May you thrive!

Thriving Beyond Surviving

Stories of resilience from a hospital chaplain

Norris Burkes

NORRIS BURKES

USAF CHAPLAIN, RET.

ISBN: 1534762973
ISBN 13: 9781534762978

This book is dedicated to my wife Becky.
After 36 years, still the best model of resilience I know.

CONTENTS

PREFACE

Two weeks after 9/11, editors at Florida Today invited me to write a spiritual response to help readers find resilience in the crisis. A month later, my newspaper column, "Spirituality in Everyday Life," was born. The column is now syndicated in nearly 40 papers nationwide. This book is a theme-based compilation of columns I've written since publishing my first book in 2006.

A word of warning: A self-described ADD author wrote this book. I skipped around when I wrote it, so feel free to read it the same way.

Please read the introduction first. After that, you may choose to read through to the final chapter or jump to the chapter of your choice. Better yet, if you find yourself uninterested in one story, restart your reading at the **bolded words that often indicate** (such as these) the beginning of the next full-length column.

Finally, to all those who have ever texted, emailed, written or left a voicemail for me:

I apologize that most of you didn't hear back from me, but please know that I've considered, read or heard all your comments, commendations and criticisms. Not one email got past me, not one message was unheard. Thank you to all my readers for making my writing dream possible.

ABOUT THE AUTHOR

Chaplain Norris Burkes has been a board-certified healthcare chaplain with the Association of Professional Chaplains since 2002. Simultaneously, he served 28 years as a chaplain in both the active-duty Air Force and the Air National Guard before his 2014 retirement.

In yet a third profession, he has been writing a spirituality column since 2001. His column offers a humorous and hope-filled approach to everyday spirituality and is syndicated in 38 papers nationwide.

He graduated from Baylor University in Waco, Texas, with a bachelor of arts in religion and journalism. He has a master of divinity degree from Golden Gate Seminary in Mill Valley, Calif. In 2012, he added a master of fine arts in creative nonfiction from Pacific University in Portland, Ore.

In recent years, Chaplain Norris has run two marathons, completing his last one in a little over five hours. Since his military retirement, he has taken up golf but says he's "not particularly trustworthy to keep accurate score."

He is the author of "Hero's Highway," about his experience in a combat hospital. He is also the author of "No Small Miracles," the father of four grown miracles and living proof that 35 years of a happy marriage is still God's greatest miracle.

CONTACT Chaplain Norris at P.O. Box 247, Elk Grove, CA 95759 or email him at comment@thechaplain.net. You can leave him a voicemail at (843) 608-9715 or find him on Twitter with @chaplain.

ACKNOWLEDGEMENTS

Thank you to editors of the newspapers that first published the stories in this book.

Montgomery Advertiser AL; Baxter Bulletin Mountain Home AK; Phoenix Sun AZ; Atascadero News CA; Elk Grove Citizen CA; Vacaville Reporter; Inside Publications Sacramento CA; Florida Today, Brevard County; The Ledger, Lakeland FL; Ft. Myers News Press FL; Journal and Courier, Lafayette IN; Star Press, Muncie IN; Courier-Journal, Louisville KY; Battle Creek Enquirer MI; Daily Press & Argus MI; Livingston Press MI; Hattiesburg American MS; The Clarion-Ledger, Jackson MS; Springfield New Leader MO: Star-Gazette, Elmira NY; Ohio Newspapers including Chillicothe Gazette, Coshocton Tribune, The News-Messenger, Fremont & Newark, Lancaster Eagle-Gazette, News Journal, Mansfield, The Marion Star, News Herald, Port Clinton, Times Recorder, Zanesville; Post and Courier, Charleston SC; The Leaf-Chronicle, Clarksville TN; The Jackson Sun TN; The Daily News Journal, Murfreesboro TN; Daily News Leader, Staunton VA and The Sheboygan Press WI

INTRODUCTION
BUILDING A THRIVING RESILIENCE

"Chaplain!" called the hospital social worker as I headed toward the parking lot. "You might not want to go home just yet."

I turned around to see her motion me closer.

"Our team is on standby tonight," she whispered. She meant our Critical Incident Stress Debriefing Team.

"Why?" I asked.

"You'd better catch the news," she said, pointing toward the television in the lobby of UC Davis Medical Center in Sacramento, where we worked. The special report conveyed the early hours of what is still the largest hostage crisis ever played out on American soil.

In April 1991, four armed robbers botched their attempt to rob a Sacramento electronics store and took hostages for human shields. They laid them on the showroom floor in front of full-length windows so the news cameras could see them. They promised to begin executing hostages if they weren't given safe passage to Thailand.

Eight hours into the crisis, police used a sniper, concussive grenades and tear gas to end it. The barrage killed three robbers and wounded a fourth, but not before the suspects killed three hostages and wounded 11 more.

The seriously wounded were taken to our trauma unit. After they received good medical care, our specially trained debriefing team encouraged them to talk about their trauma. Doing this within 24 hours of the incident was supposed to help victims quickly return to their normal lives.

With that in mind, I approached a young man who lay on a hallway gurney awaiting X-rays. I introduced myself to him and to his petite wife beside him.

As it turned out, he was a Baptist seminary student from my alma mater. We'd had the same theology professors, so I wasn't surprised when his survivor's guilt took a theological twist.

He told me that he had felt divine protection while mayhem exploded around him. He was thankful God saved him. But, he asked, "Why didn't God save everyone?"

"I don't know," I said, trying to delay his theological analysis. "I can only consider what will happen now." I was making an effort to redirect the conversation off the circular path of "why" to the more constructive question: "Where to from here?"

I wanted him to focus on his resiliency as a future minister. To do that, he had to look past this day and see a day when he'd complete his training and pursue his calling.

"Where to from here?" is the question we must all ask ourselves when tragedy strikes. What will I become from here? Will I become so mired in this tragic moment that my whole life is defined by it? Will people always know me as the guy whose home was lost in the flood? Will they always pity me as the one whose child died? Will they only remember that I was the man who was shot in the store?

The big question we have to ask ourselves when we survive such an ordeal is "Will I survive to become a person who thrives?" That is the question of this book. How can we find the faith to look past our tribulations and thrive in the future?

The student pastor would have to answer those questions on another day, because at that moment I could only hint at what was coming.

I wrapped up our conversation by asking this scripted debrief question: "What was the worst part of your ordeal?"

"The worst part was when the robber stuck a gun in my face and asked if I wanted to die," he said.

"That must be hard to hear," I reflected to his wife. She didn't answer. She simply looked at the ceiling and fainted into my arms.

Fortunately, like her husband, she was resilient. She recovered quickly and remained with her husband throughout the evening. I wasn't so lucky. I had ignored hospital training to never catch the dead weight of a fainting person. I wrenched my back and went out on sick leave for the rest of the week.

The incident served as an early example of resiliency. During my year-long internship, I counseled victims of unimaginable personal tragedies. As a chaplain, I provided a presence to people who'd been stabbed and shot as well as victims of hit-and-runs and drunk drivers. I saw healthy children die from quick-acting poison, fast-spreading cancer and ritualistic child abuse.

From the beginning of my training, I became fascinated with how the survivors of those tragedies could survive the aftermath of the heartbreaking loss of a child, the crippling of a spouse or the chronic illness that would rob them of their livelihood.

This book contains many of those stories, but it also brings insight into the journey of a hospital chaplain.

After spending that year at UC Davis, our family moved to Houston, where I took a full-time job as a professional hospital chaplain. Since then, I've spent most of my life in healthcare chaplaincy, with a few diversions into the active-duty life of an Air Force chaplain and five years as a parish pastor.

In those professions, I've walked alongside many folks who have lost more than just the wind in their sails. Many of them spent years of their life rapidly bailing their sinking boats. Others, with little chance to stay afloat, dragged to the river's bottom in a torrent of grief.

It's not only hard on them, but it's been harder on me than I would've ever imagined. It's been so difficult to hear their stories and see their consequences that I visited a psychologist last year. No, not because a few readers told me I was crazy, but as a routine part of the VA claims process.

During our 45-minute appointment, the doctor asked me to recount the trauma I'd witnessed.

I told him many of the stories I'll be telling in this book.

I told him of the days I was pastoring a Baptist church in 1989 and went to help in the tragic aftermath of Cleveland Elementary School in Stockton, Calif.

This is where Patrick Purdy shot 29 kids and killed five between 6 and 8 years old. Because of my Air Force training in mass casualties, I volunteered to deliver the unspeakable news to the parents whose children were killed.

I told him that after my years of pastoring, I became a hospital chaplain where I would see a lifetime of tragedies. As a hospital chaplain, I've waited with women as they are hospitalized through high-risk pregnancies, praying for their 30th week to bring the best chance of their baby's survival. I've waited with an agonizing father as he prays for pain medication to bring final comfort to his dying daughter.

I told him of my military life and the search-and-recovery missions I'd been on, in particular wading into Lake Okeechobee in 1999 to recover the remains of a downed Air Force pilot. We sifted through the waterborne pathogens of pond scum but found only parts of our comrade. With each discovery, someone called, "Find!" The mortuary affairs officer collected the "find" and placed the remains in a flag-draped ice chest.

The Florida weather was much like my 2005 deployment to New Orleans after Hurricane Katrina. There, I donned battle armor as I accompanied several armed patrols through the sweltering streets. Our mission was to knock down doors in search of looters, survivors and bodies.

I also recalled my time in 2009 at the Air Force Field Hospital in Balad, Iraq. I remembered a squad of three soldiers whom, despite our chaotic efforts to do everything, we just couldn't save. If we expected to lose a soldier, our chaplain team was determined that no soldier would die alone. We held the hand of each one, sitting with them until the end, no matter the hour.

But most of all, I spoke of the nearly 30 occasions I'd put on my dress uniform to drive to a town I'd never visited to deliver the news I'd never want to hear. I won't forget the home where an anguished father pounded the kitchen table as he railed against our government policies. Nor will I forget intercepting a family as they tried to go to the airport to pick up their son. He would never be coming home.

I've told these stories to the VA psychologist the same way I've told them in speaking venues all over the United States. Like the VA doctor, folks invariably ask how I'm able to recover so quickly from the horrific things that I witnessed almost daily as a hospital chaplain and combat chaplain in the Air National Guard.

This book will address many of the things that have worked for me. But truthfully, humor is one of my best tools of resiliency. I guess that's why I will often answer the question by telling the old joke about a man who resisted his wife's urging to get out of bed for Sunday church services.

"Give me three good reasons I should get out of this warm bed," he demands.

"First," she says with folded arms, "I'm your wife, and you should respect my wishes."

He doesn't move.

"Second," she says in a pious whisper, "God wants you to go to church."

No effect.

"Finally," she lets loose with the voice of a drill sergeant, "you're the pastor, and the congregation is expecting a sermon!"

As a hospital chaplain, I can relate sometimes. It happened recently as I lay in bed recalling several patients I had visited the previous week.

I thought about the nice grandmother diagnosed with a painful bone cancer. Across the hall from her was a mother who'd inexplicably died before her 12-year-old daughter could visit. Then I thought of the family of the college student who'd mysteriously drowned alone in a pool.

They were all imprinted in my mind as I lay motionless, suffering from what felt like a very cluttered soul.

Like the pastor in the joke, I started asking God for one good reason I should go to work. What do I have to offer these patients? And who am I to assure them that God is present and in control?

It's amazing how self-centered one becomes under a warm down comforter on a crisp fall morning. It's amazing how those sheets can envelop one's world.

The truth is that my world had already become pretty enveloping. As of late, I had become an undercover worrier. Nothing seemed good enough—not my writing, not my house next to the barking dogs, not my kids, not even the cafeteria food.

It had become all about me as I sang several choruses of "Me, my, mine, me."

Then I heard from God.

Not in the way televangelists hear from God; I've never heard God tell me to build television networks or prayer towers, but I do experience a guiding presence from time to time.

I sensed God telling me: "No wonder you feel inadequate. Guess what? You are inadequate. However, I'm not."

"Now," said this voice or presence, "shake yourself out of this funk and I'll guide you to someone besides yourself."

"OK, God," I prayed, "guide me to someone I can support through their troubled day. Take me beside those who are feeling alone."

As my prayer took shape, the echo of my words was enough to help me hear the message I needed to reaffirm. Namely, "The best way out of yourself is through someone else."

That is to say, God works best on our problems when we show a willingness to become the process of healing for another.

At that point, I felt a renewed awakening. So I rolled over and greeted my elementary-school-teaching wife with a kiss. "Time to get up, sweetie."

"Give me three good reasons," she said as she turned to hit the snooze button one more time.

Fortunately, this book is dedicated to giving you much more than just three reasons.

I find seven reasons to get out of bed every morning. I outlined these reasons last year when I told my wife about a modeling contest I was entering. At the time of the conversation, I was slipping into a pair of slightly skimpy running shorts.

"I didn't know your running costume qualifies you for Chippendales," she said. "So what contest are you entering?"

Let me be clear for a moment: My wife isn't funny. Sometimes my readers think she's funny. Sometimes she even thinks she's funny, but since this is a book with high standards of substantiation, for the record, she's not funny.

"Not that kind of modeling," I said. "AARP magazine is seeking contestants for its New Faces of 50+ Real People Model Search."

She seemed relieved I wasn't planning to model underwear but still wanted proof that I wasn't having a midlife crisis.

I read the AARP submission guidelines aloud that asked contestants to "...share your wisdom for living your best life at 50+ by submitting your photo and telling us just how you embrace your age."

I called my submission "Seven F-Words for My 50s," and they are now the chapter outline for this book about thriving, not just surviving.

1. Laughter. I have always kept "fun" in my agenda. I do this by watching comedies, reading comics and sharing dinnertime stories with friends. I write, read, enjoy theaters and museums, ride zip lines and attend the state fair. I do these things because fun releases natural "feel-good" hormones called endorphins. These endorphins combat stress and are therefore good for those I love and for those I serve.

2. Fitness keeps me thriving. God made us to physically interact with our world, so I embrace fitness.

I'm a runner, but I just started in 2012. I've run 10k races, half marathons and two full marathons. I started running to lose a little weight, but I continue to run because it inspires my spiritual and physical confidence. When I'm challenged by life's difficulties, running helps me go beyond what I thought possible.

When I'm not running, I play Frisbee with my dog. I go for neighborhood walks with my wife, and on holidays we hike through national parks to find waterfalls or songbirds. I swim in my pool, ride a bike down community trails and have recently learned to golf.

3. Much of my disposable income is spent on Flight. I don't really mean that I fly everywhere; I just needed an F-word to talk about travel. I'm an evangelist for travel. I work hard to reduce

my unnecessary expenses so I can divert my money toward tours, treks and trips.

I traveled to several countries as a young Air Force officer, but since turning 50, I've done so much more. I've flown to Hawaii, Alaska, Peru, Panama, Mexico, Honduras, Iraq, Australia, New Zealand, Ireland, Jordan, Ecuador and Canada. Travel helps me see that I'm not the center of the universe and that the USA has many attributes as well as faults.

When I can't afford travel, I find the water of a nearby lake, beach or waterfall. For me, water is a "God spot." Water is where I inhale the sights and sounds that renew my connection with my Creator. It's a physical place where I feel God's presence. Mostly, it's a place where I find a moment of peace and presence outside myself.

4. Finances. Yes, money helps. I'm a stickler with it. I avoid paying interest, late penalties or transaction and activation fees. My wife and I will retire on public pensions with a healthy IRA. Yes, this chaplain appreciates money.

However (and that's a huge "however"), the most precious thing money buys is time: family time; beach time; travel time. I was in my early 50s before I realized that I don't have to buy everything I want. I don't need the latest technology, the coolest cars or the largest house. Those things will count for nothing when I die. Money is to be spent on the people you love and the places that hold meaning.

5. Family. These days, "family" has multiple shades of meaning. "Family" can be an endearing term, but if you've been abused, you'll need to look for family elsewhere. You find it where you find belonging—maybe at the gym, office, church or even civic club.

My best experience of family is with my wife, children and grandchildren. I find the best meaning of "brother" in my best friend and college roommate, Roger Williams.

6. Faith. No surprise here, right? I'm a chaplain. I'm required to have faith. Well, I've known a few chaplains to lose their faith, so I never take faith for granted. Faith, like a good marriage, requires work. For me, faith is something that embraces me and keeps me from falling when all else on my list fails.

Faith is the grip the parachutist feels when his harness tightens. Faith is the grasp the trapeze artist knows as she hangs in midair only to be snatched by a skillful partner. It's a clutch that embraces you from just beyond the edge of darkness. It's an authority that knows the darkness but comes from the light. When I keep the faith, faith keeps me.

7. Forgiveness. Memorizing the Lord's Prayer is child's work. Living the Lord's Prayer is fraught with difficulty. It all seems to depend on forgiving others as we want to be forgiven. That's a pretty tough prescription, but I believe it's the most effective cure. I find my chapter on forgiveness to be my most compelling. In fact, read that chapter first if you so desire. All the chapters can be read in any order.

While these are good principles, and I've made them the basis of this book, I have to be honest about something. These principles did nothing to help me win the AARP modeling contest. It's just as well; my wife says that it's hard enough to live with a nationally syndicated columnist. She doesn't need me to become the next AARP supermodel. Just to be clear, she's not that funny.

1

LAUGH YOUR WAY THROUGH LOVE, LIFE AND LOSS

In defense of my wife, she says she's not funny because she doesn't need to be. She says that I'm funny enough for both of us—and she doesn't mean comical; she means downright goofy sometimes. She would tell you that I keep her laughing most of the time because of the ridiculously funny things that I do or that happen to me.

Laughter is the biggest factor in fun, and I'm mostly kept laughing at myself. Self-deprecating humor is the thing that keeps me going when I feel down. It's the way I recover from my mistakes, because if you can't laugh at your failures, you're just setting yourself up to become an inpatient in the psych ward.

I use self-deprecating humor because it helps me become more patient with my mistakes. I also use humor to show my readers the personal struggles of a clergy person so that the reader will better appreciate just how equal God made us all.

Unfortunately, not all of my readers see the point of my writing about personal failings in such a transparent and public way. In fact, some have written scathing letters criticizing me for the faith flubs I've dared to share.

For instance, sensuous thoughts aren't funny to everyone. Ten years ago, I wrote about the sensuous thoughts I had while getting a haircut from a female barber. An outraged reader called the hospital where I worked and left this voicemail for my colleagues to hear: "How can a 45-year-old minister have such thoughts? I thought you were a man of God. You ought to be ashamed of yourself!"

Nevertheless, I keep writing, because folks tell me they gain hope from hearing about my flops in faith. I even get positive emails from atheists and agnostics who reciprocate by sharing their struggles.

As a Christian, I believe this humor helps us relate to the human side of Jesus. In fact, as I once said in a column, "If you can't imagine Jesus stepping behind a tree to relieve himself, then you're not seeing him as human." Yup, I was buried with reproachful emails then, too.

It's this humorous side of my faith that inspired my editors to subtitle my national column "Spirituality in Everyday Life." Because, in the month after 9/11, they saw what I took for granted: namely that, if you can't find effective faith in everyday places where you live, work and die, then what good is it?

"Your humor is just plain nuts," wrote one Florida reader. She was more right than she'd dare imagine.

Case in point: When it comes to macadamia nuts, I'm a lot like Dr. Seuss' Sam-I-Am after his aversion-to-conversion experience with green eggs and ham. I can eat macadamia nuts in a box, with a fox, in a house, with a mouse. I will eat them here and there … anywhere.

Since they're also known as Hawaiian nuts, imagine my elation when I received orders to Hilo, Hawaii, with my Air National Guard unit in 2007.

My unit was participating in a two-week military exercise designed to ready islanders for problems caused by a hurricane, such as lack of communication, shelter, food, power and transportation.

It's a serious exercise, but in our evening off time, we'd often roam the town in small groups searching for good seafood.

On one particular evening, I accompanied my friends, Master Sgt. Michelle Roberts and Maj. Robert Flynn, to a beachside eatery called Harrington's. The restaurant specialized in macadamia seafood dishes and in 2009 was fittingly renamed Ponds, as the dining area sat on stilts above a koi pond.

After being seated by the hostess, Roberts and Flynn busied themselves cooing over the koi fish. However, it takes much more than multicolored fish or Hawaiian sunsets to distract me from food. I got down to business, studying the menu of macadamia-covered delights.

Eventually, the server took our orders. She promised she'd be back in a few moments with our drinks as well as some fish food to toss over the railing.

While we waited, I reopened the menu to find dessert. I quickly became distracted. Would it be macadamia cake or macadamia ice cream?

Our server reappeared and placed the drinks on the table along with what seemed like a bowl of macadamia nuts. I took a sip of Pepsi and slid a few of the golden nuggets in my mouth.

Flynn and Roberts dropped their jaws in wide-mouth incredulity; the waitress tipped her tray unsteadily.

What? I thought. Were they upset I wasn't sharing?

Suddenly, my gag reflex divulged what my friends were too shocked to say. The nutty chaplain was chomping koi food.

I retched over the railing, passing the choking chow to its intended recipients.

My companions didn't stop laughing for 10 minutes. To this day, they still laugh. To this day, I still defend myself.

"Those small food balls fit my assumptions of what a macadamia nut looks like," I tell them." I insist that they could have made the same mistake.

Honestly, my blunder reminds me of the oversight made by people who repost political commentary on Facebook or into those "Please-forward-this" emails. They push what fits their assumptions and their never-mind-the-facts viewpoint.

Like my fish food, they find stuff that confirms their political fears and persuasions. They propagate it because it confirms their dislike for a candidate or position—not because it proves anything.

This happens during every election year when politicians capitalize on our assumptions. They morph the leftover promises of "A Chicken in Every Pot" into "Change We Can Believe in" or "Make America Great

Again." All the slogans sound great because they promote what the voter assumes to be true.

Truthfully, if it wasn't for humor, especially of the self-deprecating kind, I don't think I could cope with the political world we live in. The nuts just serve to remind me that whenever someone puts an attractive platter in front of you, don't assume it's just what you need, or even what you ordered. In other words, if something seems too fishy to be true, it probably isn't macadamia nuts.

Humor is also a great coping mechanism for disappointment. Such was the case during my three-month deployment to Prince Sultan Air Base in Saudi Arabia in 1999.

I deployed to Saudi with a lot on my mind. I was anxiously waiting to see my name on the promotion list for the rank of major. For military officers, this is the most important promotion to make. If you miss it, you can't stay in the active-duty force. Simply put, missing the promotion puts your career in the toilet.

I arrived in Saudi just after Thanksgiving. Nearly twice a week, I would check with the personnel office to see if the promotion list was out. Finally, just a few days before Christmas, my chaplain supervisor, Col. Mike Bradshaw, and our staff priest, John Bell, came to my dorm room with the new promotion list.

I could tell they were carrying some news and I was excited to hear it. I felt sure their personal visit would only be good news. I figured they would have given bad news at the office, not in my room.

Bradshaw didn't know how to be subtle. Even before we sat down, he blurted the news. "You have been passed over for promotion," he said.

"You'll be reconsidered next year," promised Bradshaw. "But trust me," he said in his signature truism, "it's really a one-mistake Air Force.' You won't get another chance to remain on active duty."

For the next few weeks, my mind wasn't in the game. I felt like I was a terminally ill patient who'd been told to get his affairs in order. My life certainly felt bound for the toilet.

So I guess it was appropriate that one morning before coming to the office, I walked into the men's room to evacuate the constipated disappointment I felt. As the door closed behind me, I followed military tradition and tucked my hat into the beltline at the small of my back.

I walked into the stall and took my place on the porcelain throne, aptly labeled with the brand name "Norris." I shrugged. That's about fit for the course.

I stayed for much longer than I should have. I didn't want to go to the office. How was I supposed to be a supportive chaplain to the deployed troops when I felt so low? Finally, however, I stood to do my "paperwork."

As I discarded the paper into the receptacle, I turned to notice that some careless fool had ditched his hat in my toilet.

First, I wondered, why hadn't I previously noticed this? But my second and more sober observation was that this fool's hat had a Christian cross on it. That fool was me!

I almost cried looking at my hat in the flusher with the Christian cross affixed. Was God using a metaphor to tell me that my chaplain career was in the toilet? If so, was the military my only path of ministry? Or were there other venues? I didn't know the answer.

I had no choice but to go to the chapel office and ask our NCOIC (office manager) for a new hat.

As I unfolded my story, Master Sgt. Steve Carothers folded his 6-foot-5-inch frame in half, overcome with near stroke-inducing laughter.

He then made a comical demand. "If you want me to give you a new hat, you are going to have to give me just one good reason why I should overlook such a blame fool mistake as that."

"Well," I admitted, "there are some foolish officers in the man's Air Force. And some of them seem like they operate with a head full of crap."

He shook his head with large, agreeable nods.

"But," I said, "don't you think it takes a really good officer like myself to admit that he has a hat full of crap?"

Hearing my logic, he fell, hysterically beating the floor with his fist. "I give up, Chaplain," he declared. "You got your new hat."

The Bible says in James 5:16, "Make this your common practice: Confess your sins to each other and pray for each other so that you can live together whole and healed."

I confessed my mistake—my sin—and got a new hat. But better than that, I got a new ministry.

For you see, despite my sinking feeling that my career was flushed in the crapper of chaplain careerism, I had a creatively hysterical moment in which I emailed my hat-full story to dozens of my deployed friends.

I also happened to forward it to a Florida friend, a newspaper editor named Tom Clifford. Tom thought it was riotously funny but too inappropriate for a newspaper. Still, he saw through my "crap," and 10 months later, he invited me to write a newspaper column.

Col. Bradshaw had asked me to trust him. Trust is best left to God, not man. Now, almost 20 years after the famous toilet week, I'm winding down a long and rewarding career as a healthcare chaplain. Better yet, I've managed to finish a second career in uniform. I retired from the Air National Guard in 2014 after being promoted twice to the rank of lieutenant colonel.

If I ever meet up with Col. Bradshaw again, I'd like to tell him one thing: "Trust me, God's still not finished with me."

Most of us have some sort of irrational fear. My fear of losing my career was greatly exaggerated and seismically irrational, but it was nothing compared to my odontophobia, or fear of dentists. But as you can see, humor helps me cope.

If you met my dentist, you'd see that I really have no sane reason to fear him or his office staff. The receptionist is congenial, my hygienist a perfectionist and my dentist a consummate professional.

My anxiety is even more irrational because I have perfect teeth—no cavities, straight-arrow perfect. In fact, one dentist facetiously offered me a million dollars for them.

So what's the problem? Me.

You might say that I'm sensitive. In fact, my Air Force dental file is actually labeled "sensitive patient."

How did I earn that label?

I guess I'm a wee bit too tactile. I can't stand the scraping, grinding and pounding of the water pick. The X-ray bitewings gag me, and the polishing paste chokes me. The glaring lights blind me, and the drilling sound makes my skin crawl.

Think I'm exaggerating? Here's how my last visit went with Debbie, the new hygienist.

Me: "Can I have a blanket?"

Debbie: "Are you cold?"

Me: "No, I'm just missing my special 'blankie.'"

Debbie: Stunned.

Me: "Joking."

Debbie brings a blanket and tucks me in as if she knows the drill. Dental pun intended.

I decline her offer of safety goggles, opting for my personal pair instead. They are the darkened kind the optometrist uses when dilating your eyes. I got mine at a Utah truck stop during a summer drive through the salt flats. I save them for teeth cleaning, or in the event I'm ever asked to observe a nuclear blast.

Soon, she pries open my mouth.

Debbie: "Oh, my! How often do you brush your teeth?"

Me, through a mouthful of latex-covered fingers: "Ewey day, but I still whave whack wissues."

Debbie, withdrawing her instruments: "What?"

Me: "I have plaque issues caused by high salinity."

She brushes off my excuse and starts in with her water cannon. My feet kick the air.

Debbie, with a tender hand on my shoulder: "Are you OK?"

Me: "My regular hygienist numbs my gums."

Debbie: Skeptical stare through the glaring lights.

Me, pleading: "It's better than the laughing gas my old dentist used."

Debbie: "Oh, my. I don't think we have to go that far."

Still, ever the gentle professional, she spreads numbing gel on my gums. Instantly, it feels like an ant colony has been transplanted in my mouth.

But for the next 40 minutes, the numbing effects keep me relatively still.

Debbie: "See, that wasn't so bad. Was it?"

Me: Releasing a bad breath of incredulity.

Soon, I gather my party favor bag of floss, a toothbrush and sensitive toothpaste. I take a 15-minute decompression break in the lobby.

Truthfully, I have to give myself credit for once again facing my irrational fears.

I did that by first admitting my fear to Debbie.

After she heard my fear, we laughed our way through it. But the laughter didn't stop there. I decided to write about my fears so you could join me in laughing at myself.

As we made our next appointment, I asked Debbie how to spell her name.

Debbie: "Why?"

Me, mouth still numb: "I'm a walumnist. I'm going to make you infamous, I mean famous."

Debbie just laughs.

Note: No chaplains were harmed in this dental cleaning.

My driving can also be laughable, so if there's one place I laugh at myself, it's on the road. I've been twice stopped by police just moments after one of my speaking engagements. I suppose I was so full of myself and my oratory abilities, I wasn't even aware I was speeding.

I guess that's why I want to caution you that if you're driving during the upcoming holiday, be careful out there. The roads aren't just filled with drunk drivers.

Sometimes they're filled with reckless pastors—as they were 25 years ago in Brentwood, Calif. During the late 1980s, I was the pastor of First Southern Baptist Church in town. No, this wasn't the Southern California Brentwood of O.J. Simpson fame. This was the sleepy, rural Brentwood in Northern California where strawberries were first bioengineered.

As our town was somewhat secluded, I would often drive a few hours to attend ministers' conferences in one of the San Francisco area cities. It was on my return from one of those conferences that I found myself on the wrong end of the law.

It was about 2 a.m. one Friday when I drove into the Brentwood city limits. There were no stoplights at the time and thus little to impede my return home.

However, the town was full of stop signs.

Before I continue, let me hasten to add I was 27 years old, fresh out of seminary. With somewhat invincible thinking, I reasoned there are only Ten Commandments. To me, everything else seemed more of a suggestion.

Posted along the final half-mile homeward stretch of Walnut Boulevard were what seemed like three suggestions: stop signs about 100 yards apart.

And at 2 a.m., it certainly seemed as though a young minister, eager to return to his young bride, ought to be allowed passage through the signs at about 25 mph. Not exactly fast enough to be reckless, but fast enough to draw the attention of a fairly sleepy police officer.

In a red flash, the officer pulled me over and began to question my memory.

"Do you recall seeing the three stop signs you just blew through?"

"Yes," I said, sheepishly producing my license.

For the next several minutes, we played 20 Questions, and he quickly discovered I was a pastor.

"What church?" he asked.

"The Southern Baptist church—but probably not for long."

"Why is that?" he asked.

I reminded him the town newspaper usually published police reports, and it was difficult to imagine my parishioners reacting favorably to the news that their pastor had blown through half the stop signs in town.

As he generously wrote my ticket for running only one stop sign, he posed a question that has guided me much of my career.

He asked something like, "Have your church members never been ticketed?" In the middle of the night, the officer's question seemed to imply a church that doesn't realize it has a flesh-and-blood pastor would be a church that has long been asleep.

In the years since, I've come to realize that not only is it a sin to think of yourself as incapable of sinning, but it may be worse to think of yourself as someone who'd never want to be discovered sinning.

No, I'm not suggesting we display our sins in a way that makes us seem more human. I'm only suggesting we don't attempt to hide our sins in a way that makes us less than human. Because, as my mom always said, echoing Numbers 32:23: "Your sin will find you out."

Not long after that, The Brentwood Press published a story about speeders with a picture of an unsuspecting car driving down Walnut Boulevard.

Guess whose car just happened to be depicted with the story headlined "Walnut Boulevard Problem With Speeders."

Guilty, again.

2

FITNESS—ALIVE TO THRIVE

To be honest, I might skip this chapter if I were you. Don't get me wrong. I'm not really recommending that you skip it; I'm only saying that we hear enough grunting gurus preach their sanctimonious health sermons these days. I'm sure you can do without having to hear one from a chaplain. After all, chaplains are supposed to comfort people, right?

Well, in the event that you are not omitting this chapter, let me assure you that I won't preach. I believe we are all in the same proverbial boat and we are all trying to do better.

This chapter is simply my story of how three working principles changed my lifetime fitness. The first is the 10 percent principle. The second is the secret of showing up. The third is the power of the little bit more.

Principle #1—Change your life with a fitness tithe

With reference to my earlier driving record, I will confess that food is the only thing that will send me over the posted speed limit. When I speed, I'm usually racing the Methodists and Presbyterians to the Sunday buffet. I like food, and most of my life it's never been a problem.

In my junior year of high school, I was so skinny that I had to lie on my Air Force Academy application. Apparently there was no way to use the fill-in-the-bubble application to say that my 6-foot-1 body was 149 pounds. Despite being under penalty for perjury, I said I was 150 pounds.

So for years, I just ignored my family's obesity genes. I ate what I wanted and however much I wanted. It seemed as if God had given me a weight-gain exemption. In fact, I once bragged to a military doctor that I had a fat person inside of me screaming to get out. He actually wrote that on my medical record.

Ten years after high school, I became the pastor of First Southern Baptist Church in Brentwood. In my first few years of pastoring, I ate my way through dozens of church buffets. When the church ladies asked me what kind of vegetables I preferred, I'd often tell them they should prepare one of three kinds of vegetables: corn, corn on the cob or creamed corn. (Actually, there are three other vegetables I love: fried potatoes, scalloped potatoes and mashed potatoes.)

In quick time, I was hiding 40 additional pounds behind my pulpit. From that same pulpit, I preached against every sin but gluttony. I was good at hiding my insecurity with humor. I'd often joke that fat preachers were so common in Southern Baptist life that we consider "fat preacher" one word.

After wearing my fat suit for three years, I read an article in Reader's Digest, which suggested that altering my eating pattern by at least 10 percent would make a huge difference.

The 10 percent suggestion reminded me of the biblical notion of tithing, which is to give 10 percent of your income to the church. So I merged the idea with the biblical principle of tithing and called it my Caloric Tithe Diet. The diet was an effort to "give back" 10 percent of my calorie intake.

For instance, when I ate a cheeseburger, I'd use the dressing-soaked top bun like a napkin, discarding it onto my plate as I ate only the burger and the bottom bun.

I loved pizza, so I still slammed it down, but instead of eating my usual five pieces, I used the 10 percent rule to make my fifth piece only half size. If I went to a buffet, I reduced the second trip through the line with a smaller plate.

It was all about making such small changes that I didn't notice. It wasn't a big change. It didn't need to be. It just had to be 10 percent less than my usual diet.

In addition to incremental reductions of bad habits, I increased my good habits by 10 percent. For instance, I stopped searching for the closest parking place. I increased my walking speed by 10 percent and used elevators only when climbing more than three stories. I also ate 10 percent more fruits and vegetables.

The plan was easy enough, but the method lacked drama. So whenever I became discouraged, I reminded myself that I didn't gain the weight yesterday, so I wasn't likely to lose it tomorrow.

After nine months on the caloric tithe, I dropped 39 pounds. In fact, I lost so much weight that my doctor encouraged me to regain 10 pounds. Ironically, my habits were so well established that it took me a year to regain the 10 pounds.

At this point, you may be saying, "Nice story, but I thought this was a spiritual book, not a diet book."

If you're physically unfit, there may be a link that makes you prone to be spiritual unfit as well. For some, overeating is about trying to fill their emptiness or to anesthetize their pain.

For others, overeating is a narcissistic notion that suggests everything exists to satisfy them. For many, overeating is a futile attempt to consume the anxiety. In my case, I was I think overeating as a sensual distraction of my soul, tempting me to believe I deserve more than others.

The Bible calls this spiritual issue gluttony. Plain and simple. Gluttony was my sin, and it became a humbling reminder that no mater how thin I appear outside, there was definitely a rebellious "big boy" inside screaming to get out. That big boy is there to constantly remind me that I am a sojourner on Faith Highway and that, no matter what my current weight, I need to rely on my spiritual guide.

Principle #2—Just show up for fitness
The tithe idea worked for me for more than 20 years. I'd use it whenever my baseline weight snuck past anything more than five or 10 pounds.

However, I'll admit to a few setbacks. And when those setbacks inevitably came, I employed a principle illustrated so well in the story of Roger Revay.

I was recently reminded by my wife of that principle, when she noticed me setting our alarm for an early wake-up. She groaned in protest.

"You can blame Roger," I said.

"And Roger is…?" Becky asked.

I answered by retelling the story of Roger Revay, the patient I met while working as a chaplain at St. Joseph Hospital in Stockton, Calif.

"What brings you to our hospital?" I asked him.

"I broke my collarbone in a fall on the dance floor," he said.

I rechecked the patient notes I carried. Yes, he really was 90 years old. But even more startling, this nonagenarian expressed a single goal: to rehab his injury and return to the dance floor.

This goal seemed unrealistic in light of my anecdotal observations of elderly patients who experienced a quick decline after such a hard fall.

But Revay had taken a hard fall once before. He piloted a B-17 that was blown from the German sky in World War II on his 30th bombing mission. If anyone could return to his rug-cutting days, Roger had the right stuff.

"I remember you talking about him," my wife interrupted. "But how is he responsible for waking us so early tomorrow?"

I paused long enough to give her the stink eye before continuing my story.

A few weeks later, I had gone to see Roger at his rehab facility across town. I found him in a painful session with his physical therapist. Afterward, I asked him how he managed to survive this much pain at his age.

"Well," he said, "I just show up."

I gave him a look absent of understanding.

He explained that getting started is often the hardest point in a recovery process. So he didn't think about the pain; he only promised himself that he'd start the treatments. In other words, he'd "show up."

Wow. This classy gent was doing more than just surviving—he was thriving!

The reason Roger's story had me setting an early alarm was because my fitness program began to wane shortly after my military retirement.

After a few failed attempts to restart my fitness pledge, Roger's words took hold: "Just show up."

So I made a pledge that every Monday would become "Show-Up Monday." I promised myself that I would bury my usual excuses. I was too tired from weekend with grandkids. I had more urgent things to do. It was always either too hot or cold outside. I didn't want my early alarm to wake my wife.

I determined that I'd simply show up, put on my shorts, leash my dog, stand on the street and wait for motivation.

I did this knowing that Toby-dog wasn't going to stand still while I stared at my tennis shoes. He would start tugging us to walk. Once we started walking, Toby would start running. And once we started running, we'd run for at least 45 minutes.

My theory—or Roger's theory—was that some days, the only thing we can muster is the strength to show up. However, showing up engages the power of change. Showing up kick-starts our resiliency.

The prophet Isaiah was talking about resiliency when he said, "Those who wait upon God get fresh strength. They spread their wings and soar like eagles. They run and don't get tired. They walk and don't faint."

Those last dozen words remind me that sometimes we can only gather the strength to show up, remain conscious and not faint.

Now, 18 months later, I've renamed Show-Up Monday to something catchier: Make-It Monday. I've even calendared additional workouts I call Wake-Up Wednesday and Sunrise Saturday.

"Does Roger write your corny alliteration?" Becky asked.

"Roger doesn't have time for writing," I told her. "I called him last week. Apparently he's doing more than just showing up these days. He's going dancing every Friday and Saturday night."

My addiction is smarter than me is something I've learned from my friends in AA. Whenever I think I'm smarter than my addiction, my food addiction will always find a way. In 2008, it found that way when my scales took a drastically upward tip.

The occasion for my gain was the days leading up to my deployment to Balad, Iraq, in 2009. During the six months of preparation, I had plenty of time to eat my anxiety about leaving my family and going to a combat zone.

But it definitely got worse when I arrived to serve as the senior hospital chaplain in Balad. During my months there, I helped prepare the bodies of nine soldiers that went home under a flag. I met many other soldiers who went home without their arms or legs. The closeness to death and heartache brought an increased addiction to comfort food.

Balad was a headquarters base where 25,000 people assembled three times a day in five major cafeterias serving 24/7. The meals were big every day, but on Wednesday, we had steak, lobster and shrimp. After dinner, we walked through rows of heart-stopping dessert bars, cholesterol-clogged cheesecakes lit up in refrigerated mirrored cabinets. I usually walked out twice a day with a Baskin-Robbins milkshake.

Still, I joked about it, telling the nurses that my goal was "a pound a week."

You are losing a pound a week?" they'd ask encouragingly.

"Oh no, I'm trying to gain a pound a week."

They'd laugh with their chaplain, but it was no laughing mater. Within a few months, I'd regained all the weight I'd lost 20 years earlier.

There's nothing like serving in a war zone to bring you to terms with mortality. One afternoon, insurgent mortar fire came over our fence and hit a compound of Turkish nationals. No one died, but a dozen of them came to our hospital without feet and hands.

Later that evening, I sat in my room wondering what my family would have done if I had been one of those victims. I didn't want my children to lose their father as early as I lost mine. I'd lost my dad when he was only 65, a death he predicted.

I was only 10 years old when my father told our family that his congenital heart problem would likely cause his death within the next 20 years. His announcement prompted me to do some calculations—both mathematical and social. I already knew my times tables, so addition was easy. I would hardly be past 30 when he would likely die.

My sister presented social estimates that suggested our dad's early death wouldn't present much of a problem for us. "He'll be here for our college and our weddings," she promised. And he was.

While her assurances assuaged my immediate fears, my dad's prognosis started me thinking about how old I might be when I died. Fifty? Sixty? Or more? Would I live past that wondrous year of 2000, the date futurists predicted life would be filled with amazing things like space travel and pushbutton jobs?

Well, it didn't surprise me that I was still alive 50 years after I'd first calculated my mortality. After all, I'd managed to avoid those things emergency room staff call "risk-related behaviors." I'm a monogamous nonsmoker who wears a seatbelt and never drives while drinking.

Yet on that bunk in Iraq, I was feeling my mortality. I had relapsed, more than 20 pounds overweight. I had fallen into the old habits of eating my anxiety. Not only were these culinary habits likely to shorten my morbidity calculations, but they also constitute what the Bible calls gluttony—not exactly a favorite sermon topic of most ministers. The Baptist ministers I grew up with liked to preach on Sodom and Gomorrah and harp almost exclusively on the sexual debaucheries of the cities.

It's easy to avoid how the prophet Ezekiel quotes God's indictment of the cities for a much different kind of sin.

"'The sin of your sister Sodom was this: She lived with her daughters in the lap of luxury—proud, gluttonous and lazy. They ignored the oppressed and the poor. They put on airs and lived obscene lives. And you know what happened: I did away with them.'"

Zeke's assessment sounds very much like the pronouncements coming from America's health community. According to the National Institutes of Health, two-thirds of U.S. adults are either overweight or obese, while as many as 1 in 6 American children go to bed hungry.

The crusty old prophet was clear. Sodom is a town Americans might remember as we battle our bulge and balance our budget. Sodomites lived shorter lives, not so much because of their sexually risky behavior, but because they lived selfish, lazy and gluttonous lives without ever extending their hands to help the poor and the hungry.

The sins of Sodom reminded me that I don't want to be found simply counting down my days; I want to make my days count for myself, my family and my God.

Principle #3—Do just a little bit more

I don't think I ever realized how important it was to make every day count as I did on May 6, 2009. That was the day I returned from Iraq on a DC-10 with 180 other servicemembers. That was the day our homecoming plane made a hard landing at Baltimore/Washington International Airport. Our plane was totaled and a half-dozen soldiers were taken to area hospitals.

My idea that I'd get fit some day was overshadowed with the thought that the only day I'm ever promised is the day I'm living now. So, to the end of making every day count, I got a pound pup when I returned from Iraq.

His name is Toby, or "T-Dog" as he is known around our 'hood. He is 26 pounds of mixed ancestry whose mutt haircut favors Benji, the renowned Hollywood canine. With the long hair of a Lhasa Apso and the passion of a Jack Russell, he has the need for speed.

Since his Valentine's Day birth in 2010, he's taught me how the power of the little bit more can start you on the road to fitness. Not unlike the caloric tithe, it focuses on small improvements. The LBM, as I like to call it, is the repetitive effort it takes to make a huge change in your life over a long period of time. My discovery of the LBM first started with Toby's desire to explore the outdoors. With each venture outside, Toby pulled us to see just a "little bit more."

On our walks, we often explore a creek-side trail that splits our orderly subdivision into fraternal twins. We pause at our planned rest stop aside a community lake that spills into a wetland of malingering mallards, Canada geese and egrets. Then, we spend 20 minutes playing Frisbee. Soon, however, Toby will drag himself under a shade tree and bury his snout into the cool grass, tongue dangling.

As the weeks passed, we pushed for the extra mile to a dog park. Toby was a happy puppy for pushing himself for a LBM, because that's where he met a cute little Jack Russell named Mia. They chased balls, begged for treats and tore the grass under their paws with quick moves. Eventually, our walks morphed into slow jogs together. As Toby grew, my 37-inch waist began to shrink. As Toby got faster, I got faster.

Six months later, I lined up on a college track to take my annual Air Force fitness test. The course was six laps, 1.5 miles. If I couldn't make it in less than 15 minutes, disciplinary letters from my commander would start the process of ending my military career.

Thirteen minutes and 30 seconds later, I finished my last lap with a two-minute improvement on my best previous time. Toby had done his job. The LBM had made all the difference.

I have a smart dog, but even Toby has limits. Eventually, Toby became exhausted at my attempts to push him just a LBM. So, after a few miles, I'd bring him home, sit him in a front of a water bowl and go off for another few miles. By the end of the year, I was pushing my running routine into six-mile runs, shaving still another inch off my waist. I was finally feeling the runner's high I'd heard so much about. My family thought I was looking more like Run-Forrest-Run from the 1994 movie "Forrest Gump."

Late in 2012, I did an eight-mile run. It felt so good, I came home to announce that I would register for a half marathon. Toby just stared at me from his empty food dish and allowed my wife to speak for him.

"Are you crazy?" she asked.

When friends and family asked me if I thought I could really run that many miles, I admitted, "I don't know." But, I'd quickly add, "I only know that last week, I ran eight miles, and this week I'm doing a 'little bit more.'"

As each month passed, I ran past eight miles, then nine and then 10 miles. Life felt good. I'd lost 25 pounds, I was writing my second book and, at 54, I still had comb-able hair. In short, I was feeling on top of my warped and wobbly world.

Then my wife introduced me to Eva Nelson, a teacher colleague from our church. After a few minutes of church chat, Eva mentioned her recent half marathon runs and challenged me to race with her team.

Unfortunately, my male ego sometimes trumps my chaplain card. "Eva is only five years younger than me," I reasoned. "I should be able to do anything a 'girl' can do." So, in that altruistic vein (or, perhaps, vain), I paid my registration for the American River Parkway run in Sacramento.

For the next six weeks, I joined Eva's running group, called Running For Rhett. The group was started by Beth and Randy Seevers, whose son Rhett was born with severe cerebral palsy in 1997. Beth and Randy were parents of three other children and worked tirelessly to make a life for all of them. Yet, tragically, Rhett died unexpectedly on March 13, 2004.

On the first anniversary of Rhett's passing, a friend introduced Beth to her first half marathon. During the next two years, she enlisted others to run alongside her until, on Dec. 7, 2007, friends and family founded the Runnin' for Rhett nonprofit foundation.

Their mission is to "Let Rhett's story inspire, uplift and encourage all to move into life." And while not everyone in the group has such a tender story as the Seeverses, most of them do have a story in which they are "born again" after bad health, careers or relationships.

They pursued the scriptural admonition to "Put everything out of our lives that keeps us from doing what we should." Let us keep running in the race that God has planned for us.

And that's exactly what this team did during this half-marathon: They followed the course and they kept running the race. They sustained encouragement for themselves, for me, the newbie, and for the teammate who kept losing her stomach contents.

Finally, at 12.9 miles, when I still couldn't see the end of the road, I had one question: Did some joker move the finish line? I was expecting to see it five miles back. At 2:34:18, but still 30 minutes behind Eva's best time, I bolted across the finish line.

A few minutes later, I found Eva sipping a Coke. "So, are you ready to register for a marathon now?" she asked me.

As crazy as it sounded, both Eva and Toby had me thinking it just might be possible. I kept asking myself, what could be possible if a person was willing to do just a little bit more than the day before? And a little bit more after that? Maybe "impossible" is just an arbitrary word.

What kind of changes might we see if we added one more minute of prayer to our daily meditation?

Or what might happen if we added another five dollars to our monthly charity contributions and then another five dollars each month after that?

What would it be like if we learned the name of one passerby? Get acquainted with one more co-worker or one more churchgoer? Then after that, another.

You see where I'm going here? There's power in Toby's LBM formula.

Of course, Jesus characterized the little-bit formula long before Toby did, but Jesus called it faith.

He compared the little-bit idea to the mustard seed when he said that the seed is "… the smallest of all seeds, yet when it grows, it is the largest of garden plants…."

This week, I challenge you to exercise your faith as well as your body. Exercise and push to add one more good thing in your life. As far as marathons go, I registered for the California International Marathon and promised my wife that it would be my one more good thing.

While the chow line in Iraq had helped me gain weight, seven months of Runnin' for Rhett gave me a 97.5 percent on my fitness test, placing me in the top 10 percent of Air Force personnel. At 175 pounds, I was shopping for a new swimsuit because the old one kept falling down. Wow, I know that's not a picture you expected in a spiritual book.

When race day came, so did two inches of predicted rain. Only 6,474 of the 9,300 registered runners even bothered to show up. But the Rhett team all showed. At 7:45 on a Sunday morning, I wobbled toward the start line to begin a 26-mile run through a blistering rainstorm that was flooding the lower parts of Sacramento. The 40-mph wind gusts chilled me in places I can't talk about here, but I was starting to believe what most of my friends, including my dear, sweet wife, Becky, had been telling me: "You are absolutely crazy!' "

I was on the start line dressed as our coach had advised, donning a cutout plastic garbage bag over my slick running clothes. When I added military prescription goggles, I resembled a roadside panhandler more than a serious runner.

With 13-13 as my running number, I felt a tinge of superstition. I was nursing a strained calf muscle and a recently developed cough, but I was hoping to dismiss both with anti-inflammatory drugs and cold medications.

More than crazy, I felt a chill of fear. I was afraid I wouldn't finish. I was afraid I might get hurt. I was afraid of the dark, the rain and the cold. I was afraid I'd disappoint my family who had missed my attention during the weeks of training.

As we stood waiting for the start, my running buddy, Eva Nelson, laid a hand on my shoulder. Becky and I know Eva and her husband, Scott, from our church. That's where Eva had "guilted" me into running the marathon.

Water was pouring off our billed running hats when Eva launched into a coaching pep talk that naturally morphed into a prayer for courage and strength. When she was done, I think we both felt dampness in our eyes that wasn't all attributed to the rain.

We patted each other on the back one more time and started the race on an 11:30-minute-per-mile pace with a dozen running buddies from Runnin' for Rhett. We'd trained at that pace for a few months, and most of us were confident we could maintain it.

Very quickly, the race became fun as we joked, splashed and even sang song snippets like "Raindrops keep falling on my head" and "The sun'll come out tomorrow." Eventually, the rain stopped after three hours.

At five hours and 38 minutes, my gelatinous legs propelled me across the finish line and into sunny downtown Sacramento. I have to say that while my pace lagged, my course stayed true, my fears were vanquished, my courage renewed and my strength sustained. And I'd more than survived.

3

THRIVING THROUGH TRAVEL

The third of my seven F-words is flight. No, I don't expect you to sign up for flight school or strap on a hang glider and jump from a cliff. I use the word flight to force a connection to the word I really want to use: Travel.

I relate travel to resiliency for three reasons. First, it gives you a new perspective. As clichéd as it may seem, it really will broaden your horizons when you see the different ways people live. Second it will help you develop the resolve you need for life as you overcome the obstacles that traveling presents. But mostly, I encourage people to travel because it takes you out of your comfort zone and helps you dismantle the ethnocentricities that often blind us all to our cultural privileges. In other words, you'll see how people the world over are seeking many of the same things from life.

If you want to thrive and not just survive, you'll find that travel teaches you some crucial lessons in resiliency. I believe this to be so true that I'll often ask the patient facing a terminal diagnosis things like, "Do you have any place you've wanted to go, but have never gone? Have you left anything undone or unsettled?"

These are the types of questions that were haunting Bob, the music minister in the church I pastored in 1981. Bob had a lot of things he wanted to do when he retired, but mostly he'd always wanted to see the United States from a recreational vehicle. He'd delayed those plans all his life until, on his 65th birthday, he and his wife Maria bought an RV. A few weeks later, our church members saw them drive out of the little town of Hopland, Calif., headed east to Ohio.

A month later, I received an early-morning phone call. The caller's voice was trembling. It was Bob.

"She's gone."

"What? Who? How do you mean?" I asked groggily.

"My wife," he said.

Through his sobs, I heard him explain he'd been driving on the interstate when he and his wife began to argue about something insignificant. Things got angry and tense. Suddenly, she turned to him and said, "I'm going home."

"Go ahead," he said, not knowing exactly how she meant that.

Then, in one terrifying instant, she opened the door and slid herself onto the road at 60 mph.

A postmortem exam revealed that Maria had undiagnosed brain tumors that caused her thinking to go awry. Her life really ended long before she knew it. They had both waited their entire life to seize their day— then, suddenly, it was gone.

Much like this couple, there were two revolutionaries in the Easter story who always wanted to seize their day and change their world but somehow never got around to doing it. We meet them as they hang on crosses, dying on each side of Jesus.

One man ridicules Jesus, but the other hints that he'd never taken the time for a spiritual road trip. Perhaps he'd hoped to find a truer path for his life than dying for a meaningless cause.

But thankfully, in his last few life breaths he expressed a desire to find a more spiritual path. With that request, Jesus granted him a road trip to paradise.

Talk about networking. This guy finally was in the right place at the right time.

Yet you have to wonder how this man had spent his life.

Had he spent it always wondering about spiritual things? Had he delayed the spiritual journey because it wasn't the right time in life? It was a wonderful miracle that Jesus was there to stamp his paradise passport, but what might his life have been like if he'd started his journey much earlier?

Spiritual road trips are sometimes expensive, but the cost of staying home is almost always a deflated life. It is easy to live life with the ambiguity of the "someday," but there is a time when you must give your final answer. There is a moment when you must decide to take your life out of the "always-wanted-to" category and place it into the "done" category.

To move into the done category, I believe you must ask yourself the same question I've asked many terminal patients. What do you want to do before you die? What do you want to see before you die? Or what is it that you need to settle in your life?

Whatever it is, I've found many of those answers for myself in travel.

Many of you may be saying the same thing readers often tell me when I write about travel in my syndicated newspaper column. "That's nice, Norris, but not everyone is so privileged. Not all of us can afford to buy a domestic airline ticket, much less an international ticket."

I get it. I really do. Chaplains make less money than even the school-teacher I married. In fact, much of our travel was paid for by the military or through my daughter's travel benefits with Alaska Airlines. But even when travel wasn't free, I always made it a priority.

Staycations count as travel, too. Whenever plane travel wasn't possible, I'd employ one of four techniques to help me widen my worldview.

- Read books, but not just travel books. Read nonfiction about history, religion, cuisine and culture, and include international fiction like "The Kite Runner." Get "Reading Lolita in Tehran" or works by the increasingly popular Turkish writer Orhan Pamuk. These books offer Middle Eastern views that have been hidden by war.
- Mix with people from other cultures and countries. Ask your Afghan neighbor to describe life in his country. Get your Sikh veterinarian to talk about his religious holidays. Turn a chance meeting with a Russian barber into an explanation of Russian politics.

If you are really daring, visit a Muslim mosque or Sikh temple to find that it's not so daring after all.

- My personal favorite is to try cultural food. Go to a food festival sponsored by a Greek Orthodox or Buddhist congregation or share a meal in a Baha'i temple. In my travels, I've eaten everything from rattlesnake and alligator to kangaroo burgers and guinea pig meat. Food is a wonderful test of your ethnocentric taste buds.
- Visit local nature sites. Nearly everyone lives close to some wonderful part of God's creation. Looking at nature humbles me. It reminds me that there are as many forms of beauty in nature as there are in people. Recently, my wife Becky and I were able to combine local trips with beauty and entertainment. The experiences helped us rediscover the spiritual renewal possible in local travel.

Interstellar travel can be as close as your own backyard. No worries, I'm not talking about a space shuttle trip. (But, just to set the record straight, I would like to be the chaplain for the first Mars mission.)

Nonetheless, if you've read much of my newspaper column, you'll know that while I'm pretty starry-eyed about my wife, I also get starry-eyed about God's world, too. And August is my chance to combine both loves.

That's when the city of Reno hosts its famous Hot August Nights, the largest classic car event in the United States. By car, Reno is less than three hours through the Sierra Nevada mountains from our Sacramento home.

When we arrived, we spent our afternoon eating fair food and looking at old cars. Since Becky's a crooner fan, I popped for tickets to the Frankie Valli tribute show. After the show, I was contemplating our next entertainment venue when my smartphone calendar pinged a reminder of the annual Perseid meteor shower.

Near penniless from the overpriced casino show, I saw the reminder as divine direction. After all, the annual shower has entertained earthlings for at least 2,000 years. So we ditched the dimming wannabe starlets and the manmade lights of "The Biggest Little City in the World," grabbed our dog from the hotel and drove 20 minutes southwest to a trailhead on Mt. Rose.

We stopped our truck and stepped into near total darkness. We waited only a few minutes and God sent our first meteor to scratch the night sky. We stood for a moment with the giddiness of celestial prospectors, then scurried into our truck bed, wrapped ourselves in blankets and posted our puppy for guard duty.

During the next 75 minutes, we watched pebble-sized icy droplets rip the heavens open like a zipper. We counted 50 of the little sky scratchers as they drew straight lines across the moonless sky at a perky 18 miles per second. It was as if God was busy sketching architectural plans for another universe.

This was interstellar travel found not far from our ZIP code. We "ah'd" and "ooh'd"and "whoa'd" like children watching a circus act, and at times we jumped in startled wonder as if we'd had an ice cube dropped down the backs of our shirts. We had spent our day wowing classic cars, savoring delicious food and humming the oldies, but nothing man-made matched the stunning show God gave us by flicking frosty slivers across the night sky.

At the end of the day, I couldn't say that God had skipped fiery rocks across the sky as a personal message just for us, but I can say that there was something to be heard that night. For even though the streaks were silent, my wife and I spoke only in whispers as if fearing that somehow we might not be able to hear God's voice. Even Toby-dog was quiet.

"Does God really talk to you, Chaplain?" you may ask.

No, not in audible tones. But I must say in our mountaintop moment, nothing ever sounded so sacredly wonderful. It was as if I could hear the planets spin, as if I could hear myself aging, and as if I could hear the clouds greeting each other. I held the hallowed moment in my heart and heard the scripture "Be still and know that I am God."

We'd started the evening hearing the Frankie Valli singers croon "Oh What a Night," but it was God who made sure that it was!

"Does God have a place on the coast?" was the question I recently considered. I discovered the answer is yes. I know because I've been lucky enough to spend my entire life within a few hours of coastal communities in Florida, California, Texas and even Turkey.

I'm not alone in my love for the coast. As a minister, I often hear people say that they can worship God at the beach as easily as a church.

So I recently decided to head to the beach to see if God indeed had beachfront property. It had been one of those weeks when the inconsistencies of my faith had been apparent to more than just myself. It was one of those weeks when I was longing to simply be the same person I had been the previous week.

As I parked my car beachside, I told God the ground rules. "I just need a moment to double-check stuff with you—a moment to make sure you're still covering my back. So I thought I'd say howdy here at the beach. I know that you make every day special, but I'm needing this day to be extra."

So, on the water's edge, I found an isolated rock and quickly breached its top. Sitting atop the rock with my soul exposed, I began searching the waves for some kind of epiphany. As I searched, the cold wind seemed to pound my heart like a burglar's hammer hoping to unlock a treasure and I hid my face beneath my sweatshirt's hood.

From this rock, I was hoping to find a still place, a place where I could both hide and be exposed, see and be seen—a place high enough to make my prayer heard but low enough to nurture humility.

My prayer began:

> Lord, find what I've hidden
> Touch what I've hurt
> Open what I've closed
> Teach what I wouldn't learn
> Fill the places I've emptied
> And empty what consumes me.
> Release what I've captured
> Hold what escapes me
> Invade what I defend
> And defend what I've surrounded
>
> Amen

I opened my eyes, watched the sun set across the waves and easily concluded, "Wow! God really does own beachfront property!"

As I climbed off the rock, I noticed my children writing messages in the sand. And like an Etch A Sketch turned upside down, the messages in the sand were quickly rinsed away in the finicky waves.

It was a metaphor that I saw my pastor re-enact the next day in church.

While church is usually a more traditional place to seek God, my pastor often works outside of tradition. That Sunday morning, he'd brought a tub of sand and placed it on the altar. During Communion, he challenged us to come and write in the sand the thing that we feel separates us from being the person that God created us to be.

So, there in the dimly lit altar of sand, I imagined myself back on the beach. I saw myself climbing off that rock, and in my heart's imagination I could feel the water flush my shoes with frozen tickles. I felt myself sloshing through wet sand, clouding the water where I walked.

Still meditating on the pastor's challenge, I saw myself come to the wet sand where the waves swept every third wave or so. There, I wrote the thing that seemed to separate me so often from God.

Now, standing amid several others who'd come to the altar, I wrote the word "Self."

Then, as quickly as I'd written it, the pastor told us to smooth over it. "As scripture promises," he told us, "God erases our failures. God stands ready to separate us from our failures as 'far as the east is from the west.'"

Wow, God had a residence here in my sandy church as well. On the previous day, I had encountered God on a rock. Now on this Sunday, the rock on the beach had moved to my place in the pew.

It's easy to find rocks. What's hard about rocks is figuring out what to do with them.

Will we hide under them? Will we proclaim from them? Will we fight to defend them? Will we throw them?

Or will we use them as touchstones to a higher place where we can see beyond ourselves? My guess is that sacred ground can be found in many places. Sometimes God finds us in Sunday hymns. Other times, God finds us in the seaside winds.

Travel brings thriving resiliency. I believe in the benefits of travel so much that if someone gave me free airline tickets, I wouldn't ask where we're going until the flight attendants finished preflight instructions. I think that's pretty much how my family and I ended up stationed in Turkey for two years. I simply told my commander that I wanted to see the world, and he made that possible.

After that, the military gave me more airline tickets to places like New Orleans for the Katrina cleanup, Saudi Arabia for Operation Southern Watch, Iraq for Operation Enduring Freedom and the jungles of Panama for Operation New Horizon.

The best free travel ticket I ever got was my return trip from my deployment to Iraq. This was one of those occasions when travel can help you build the resolve you need in overcoming obstacles in life. It can help you bounce back after a particularly debilitating event. In fact, bounce is a great word to describe the plane I was on as I returned from my Iraq deployment on a chartered World Airways DC-10 in 2009.

Our plane made a drastic bounce on the runway. Security cameras recorded a large puff of smoke, and eyewitnesses would tell FAA investigators that they thought the plane was going to flip. A second bounce delivered an estimated 3.2 Gs, and plastic ceiling molding fell on us as oxygen generators swung like piñatas. Several seat backs snapped backward while passengers along the left windows watched the yellow centerline and I watched our wing drift over the grass.

We sailed back into the air as the cockpit voice recorder captured pilot Craig Gatch asserting: "8535 heavy declaring an emergency go-around."

When we regained some altitude, my fellow passengers spoke in muffled voices. No one wanted to be the first to cry, but clearly no one wanted to die without protest. Some were praying or holding hands or just staring at their feet.

I rested my forehead on my seat back to pray, even as I wondered if I heard a judgmental voice in it all. My shortcomings felt as though they were being weighed on the scale of a spiritual assayer. Was there a deity somewhere with a one-piece eyeglass assessing my life with a doubtful squint?

Had I been a good husband and dad? Or had I been too absent, physically and spiritually? Was it OK to feel scared? Or should I gather my wits and start a rousing chorus of "Amazing Grace"?

I kept praying, spending the next few minutes asking God, "What about all these passengers?" A soldier was about to meet his new son for the first time. An airman was trying to make a marriage work again. They all wanted another chance. Would they have it?

In a center aisle seat, catty-corner from me, a young officer was wiping her tears. I stretched across the aisle to offer my hand as a reminder she wasn't alone. I wanted to hold it until we landed, but the awkwardly angled reach caused me to break loose and join her hand with the chaplain assistant sitting beside her.

As we approached the airport again, the flight attendants told us to grab our ankles and lower our heads. Then the pilot added his instruction to "brace for impact!" But instead of impact, we landed as calmly as if we were sailing across a mountain lake.

Slowly we looked up from our crash/prayer position and started clapping like we had never expected another tomorrow.

Before we deplaned down portable stairways, five people were removed for medical care, including the first officer with a broken back. Behind us, debris littered an unusable runway.

Few of us could make much sense of the incident. Many would say to me things like, "Chaplain, we expected to die in Iraq, but never in Baltimore."

Investigators declared the plane a total loss, saying the main spar (the structural member that supports the wings while the plane is grounded) was broken. This meant our pilot literally risked losing our wings during his 10-minute go-around. But I suppose that's the true meaning of "flying on a wing and a prayer."

I came home from that trip a bit shaken about flying and traveling. Nevertheless, I took many more plane trips when I accepted speaking invitations from the towns where my newspaper column was running during my deployment.

"I've Been Everywhere, Man" is the Johnny Cash hit that I often sing on my travels. In the years after my crashing homecoming, I've sung the song all the way to San Diego, Denver, Las Vegas, Seattle, Charleston, upstate New York and several cities in Florida, Arkansas and Ohio.

Because I often fly on an airline that doesn't assign seats, I developed a strategy for finding the best seat. Unfortunately, sometimes the strategy fails me, as it did some years ago when I took the last available seat: a middle seat over the wing. As the plane began its ascent, the sun bounced off the wing directly into my eyes.

"Excuse me." I asked my seatmate. "Would you mind lowering your window shade?"

Looking up from her travel magazine, she proclaimed, "I got this seat for the view. Sorry."

It was a pretty abrupt response to my polite request. I found it unbelievable how anyone might consider an airfoil to be a picturesque view. I wondered if there might possibly be a way I could convince her that it was in her best interest to close the shade.

First I took the biblical high road. Since the Bible commands Christians to "pray for those who spitefully use you," I said a silent prayer. I'll admit I had mixed motives. I was praying that I'd calm down, but I was also secretly hoping that the sight of me burying my face in my palms might intimidate her into closing the dang shade.

That didn't work. I had another thought. I sometimes can get a sneezing fit when exposed to bright sunlight, so for a brief moment, I considered staring into the glaring sun. I figured that if that promoted me to sneeze, she'd close the shade. Then I'd apologize, call it a baptism and hand her a towel.

I didn't do it, though. I couldn't. God bless me. However, I did think about evoking a sneeze by pulling a nose hair. Didn't do that either.

You needn't say it. I know I was being petty. I prayed harder. "Forgive me, Lord, for thinking such terrible things. Amen."

Nothing. No change in attitude. My prayer failed to restore my spiritual equilibrium—quite the opposite, really. I thought of more things I could do. I reached for the airsickness bag and played with it a moment, wondering if I ought to recall the famous Clint Eastwood line, "Hey, lady, do you feel lucky?"

I leaned back and looked at the ceiling. "I'm sorry, God. Travel can sure bring out the jerk in me sometimes."

No worries, though. Being a jerk can be a legitimate part of our faith journey. After all, even the Apostle Paul could be a jerk. After his blinding conversion to Christianity, Paul said he still found himself entangled with less than perfect attitudes. In Romans 7:19, Paul wrote, "For the good that I want, I do not do, but I practice the very evil that I do not want."

Occasionally I get a letter from someone who believes that my short-comings, such as the ones on the plane, "are not to be excused in the clergy." The truth is that, if all my sins were lined up end to end, there'd be enough to build a stairway to heaven—or maybe even a stairway to the hot basement place.

The plane event became just another way in which we bring our un-holy intentions into plain events. However, if we choose to approach these irritations as moments to remember God, they can serve as a reality check on how we travel in this world. Those realizations are called "progress." In the end, I realized that it is not my ability to be perfect but my ability to confess my imperfections to a forgiving God that makes me such a fre-quent flyer in God's Grace.

Fortunately, I'm not always such a pain to my seatmates. Sometimes I'm actually helpful.

It was a plain plane conversation I began some years ago with a man seated next to me on a cross-country flight. You know the type. What do you do? Where are you from? Yada yada yada. I told him I was a pastor, and of course the conversation slowed abruptly.

As we neared our destination, the pilot disrupted our banter with something you don't want to hear your pilot tell you at 30,000 feet. "We have a slight problem. You have noticed that we've been circling our air-port for the last 15 minutes because an indicator light is telling us that our nose landing gear might not be down."

The pilot's announcement jump-started my conversation with my seat-mate. Suddenly this stranger began telling me how he'd let his family and his spiritual life slip away during his climb up the corporate ladder. The man wondered aloud if there would ever be a time when he could renew that spiritual connection.

"Why not renew it now?" I asked.

"Now? Here on the plane?" he asked.

"Yes," I said. "God isn't a bit embarrassed."

He told me he'd think about it, and we both let conversation migrate elsewhere.

After we'd finished our last peanut bag, the co-pilot walked through the cabin, pulled up a section of the aisle carpet and looked into the belly of the plane. A few minutes later, the pilot came back on the PA to say that the co-pilot reported that the landing gear did appear to be down.

"However," he added, "we have no assurances that the gear is actually locked into position, so we will have emergency vehicles meeting us on the runway." And with that, the flight attendants reviewed our party favors like oxygen masks and escape slides.

The attendants gave the signal to lean forward in a crash position. As we came within a hundred feet of the runway, I saw an armada of emergency vehicles whizzing along. A few minutes later, we slowed for an uneventful stop. The turbines softened and the clapping started.

My fellow passenger turned to me and asked if I thought there was some sort of higher purpose in the two of us traveling together.

I'd like to tell you that I gave him a sage answer, but I was too busy rooting through my carry-on to replace my sweat-soaked shirt. Most of my answer was simply a nervous laugh and "Yeah, well, maybe."

When my wife met me at the gate, we hugged just a bit tighter as she asked about the fire trucks.

"They came to meet our plane," I said.

She bounced a look off me that went into the next county. The thought that she'd nearly seen my plane cartwheel through the local rice fields brought some fairly instant tears between us.

Years have passed since that incident, and I can't tell you if my seatmate ever found a "purpose" for that little scare.

The only purpose I can tell you is that it helped me see how limited my life really is. It reminded me how I'd been living my youth straining to make my future but not thinking about the present I was living in today.

When you're young, you can spend a great deal of time living in the future. You want to ride along with Johnny Cash and go everywhere, man.

When you're old, you tend to spend too much time living in the past, trying to convince everyone that you really have been everywhere, man.

And the problem with living at the address of Future or Past is that there is never a way to relive the past, and my plane ride assured me that I can never be confident of the future.

So these days, as much as I can, you can find me right here in the present. And as far as I can see, that was the plain purpose of that plane ride.

The Pillow Flight is what I call the early flight that often leaves at zero dark thirty. I call it that because I always carry my most important tool for travel resilience: my pillow.

Recently, as I stooped to kiss my sleeping beauty and grab my pillow, I failed to notice the pillowcase she'd put on it the night before. It wasn't until I arrived inside the well-lit terminal that I realized the color of the pillowcase: bright pink. It's not that I'm sexist. I truly think real men can wear pink, but a pink pillowcase is crossing some sort of manly boundary, and I have boundary issues.

You're probably surprised a grown man who openly carries a pillow would be concerned with something so inconsequential as the color of his pillowcase.

But I was.

Annoyed I'd been exposed for my pink, I sideswiped my way down the moving sidewalk unit. I came upon a girl sucking her thumb and swinging her baby doll. The girl pointed to me, and her mother responded to her in a whisper.

Was it my pillow? Was she making fun of it? Hmm. Maybe she wanted it. I quickened my pace.

Hoping no one at the security checkpoint would notice the downy softness of my pillow, I slung it on the conveyor belt. Truthfully, they wouldn't have noticed it if I hadn't nearly forgotten it on the receiving end.

"Wait," the security lady yelled. "Is this your pink pillow?"

I'm certain people were suitably horrified. I felt like the security guard was going to demand to see my man card.

As I reached for it, she smiled in that perfectly sassy way of someone who's got you in the crosshairs of humiliation and said, "You'll need this for night-night."

Truth be told, my fellow travelers weren't so much staring at me as they were staring beyond me—beyond me to their own problems and their own embarrassments.

They were remembering the times when they'd hauled their own shame into a public place, the times in which they were shown to be someone less than they imagined themselves to be.

Those exposing moments usually come as we encounter life's little security checkpoints. These checkpoints usually materialize in the places where it becomes important to strip us of those items that give us comfort or false importance.

Just as at the airport checkpoints where you lay aside the entrapments of importance (cellphones, fat wallets, Rolex wannabes, designer shoes and, yes, even pink pillows), there are divine checkpoints where we encounter God, who can thoroughly search our souls.

They are the places that tend to strip us of our self-interest, our pride, our hardness, our excuses and our grudges. I find my checkpoints in the hospital chapel, where I often will ask God to sound an alarm if I'm carrying stuff that I shouldn't be carrying.

Sometimes I find these checkpoints on the beach, where I can almost hear the waves laughing as they witness the grandiose image I've constructed of myself.

Life will nearly always present these serendipitous checkpoints. They will be checkpoints we can anticipate with great expectation. For at these places, we can be sure God always will sound the gawking buzz to tell us we've been found out.

And with that, I'll pull my pink pillow up to my travel beard and say, "Night-night, y'all."

Now, would you all please join me in the second verse of "I've Been Everywhere, Man"?

Bucket list is a phrase popularized in the 2007 movie by the same name. The phrase conveys things people would like to do or see before they kick the proverbial bucket. I believe, as the movie portrayed, that planning and financially saving for big trips give me inspiration to push myself further in both miles and in life.

Making such a list helps you postpone your inevitable bucket kicking. So I put two places on our bucket list of travels. These places brought me to such a humbling encounter with God's creation that I encourage everyone I meet to go there. The first bucket trip was a 12-day cruise bound for parts of Australia and New Zealand.

The occasion was our 30th wedding anniversary. It was a very busy cruise. In Sydney, we visited the world-famous Blue Mountains, where we rode the steepest railway in the world, descending 1,350 feet through a cliff-side tunnel into an ancient rainforest.

In the city of Hobart, Tasmania, we cuddled with koalas, hand-fed kangaroos and found ourselves bedeviled by the Tasmanian devil as it devoured a chicken carcass.

In New Zealand, we toured the Te Puia cultural center for the indigenous people of New Zealand called the Maori. The Maori came to New Zealand from Tonga and Samoa in canoes between 800 and 1,350 ago.

Adjoining the cultural center was the renowned Pohutu geyser. It is one of only five geysers in the world with regular eruptions. The eruptions shot to such a height that the trees in the background were hidden from view.

We spent five days in New Zealand but saved the best for our last day.

In Waipoua Forest, we stood as specks before the most massive of all life in New Zealand. Its kauri trees have roots in the Jurassic age.

Standing under a tree named the Tane Mahuta (The Lord of the Forest), we looked up nearly 60 feet before we saw a branch.

My first reaction was a sucking gasp. It was the sound of credulity leaving my body. I can't come close to describing it. It was one of those unique moments that God gives us when we are again reminded that we aren't the center of our universe. There are bigger things more magnificent than man could make. This was indeed one of God's special temples. It was one he created long before man could erect a steeple, a minaret or an ark.

I humbly felt what Job may have felt when rhetorically asked where he was when God declared the boundaries of the sea.

"Who took charge of the ocean when it gushed forth like a baby from the womb?" God asked.

Job was smart enough to remain silent.

"That was me!" God declared. "Tell me if you know so much."

Speechless, I lay down on my back, atop roots hundreds of years old, below branches a few hundred feet above that stretched a hundred feet across. Twenty-one time zones away from my own, I'd found some synchronicity with the awesome creative power of God.

A few days later, I was back in the United States attending traditional worship and singing familiar songs in a place made from mortar and wood. The truth is that I barely carry a tune in a bucket. However, I do hope that I'll never forget the tune I carried out of the New Zealand forest. It was a place that I was glad made my bucket list.

Our second bucket list trip took place five years later to the Galapagos Islands. It was there my wife, Becky, and I had an unforgettable encounter with a booby of the blue-footed variety.

We were two of 10 tourists on a four-day cruise through four of the beautiful islands that sit 600 miles off the humid Ecuadorian coast. This was the place where Charles Darwin found many of the icons of biological evolution. He found them here, not just surviving but thriving as the fittest in their group. Twice a day, crew members helped us into an inflatable dinghy and steered us ashore. Our island guide took us down strictly controlled, narrow trails through habitats teeming with turtles, iguanas, sea lions, crabs and numerous varieties of birds.

On the third day, we disembarked onto the island my birder wife had been anxiously awaiting: the rocky shore of North Seymour. For the next two hours, we wound through large colonies of nesting frigates and blue-footed boobies. Becky lost her teacher demeanor, quickly becoming a wide-eyed student of everything she saw.

Suddenly, she pointed toward a tree and said, "I think that booby is dead."

We all turned to see a booby hanging, blue feet up, while the guide grabbed his binoculars.

"No way that bird should be in that tree," he said.

"Why?" I asked, being a bit of an ornithological booby myself.

"Those webbed feet aren't built to land on branches."

"Looks like he's impaled those giant feet onto the tree thorns. However," he said, bringing the bird into sharper focus, "he's still alive!"

We were stunned to hear it, but not as stunned as we were when he asked for a volunteer to help rescue the bird.

"Take Becky," I said, inspiring a quick group concurrence.

For the next several minutes, our group shared the binoculars and watched Becky and our guide attempt to disentangle the booby. Eventually they were able to remove it from its impalement and place it on the ground where it would recover or die.

When we returned to our ship, I lay my seasick self down in our tiny cabin to contemplate the booby who'd paid the price for flying into a place he didn't belong, for trying to gain something that wasn't his.

The moment inspired this confessional prayer:

Lord,

There are times when I'm tempted to fly into places I don't belong, tempted to swoop in to claim a territory not meant to be mine.

There've been times when I've entered into personal arguments that aren't mine, and I've offered opinions that weren't sought and made judgments that were uncalled for.

Like the feckless booby, I've sought nourishment from barren and thorny sources. While making a seemingly stealthy landing, I've only impaled myself on the consequences of being where I shouldn't.

Forgive me, Lord, for the times when I've called out for rescue from those places, somehow hoping that redemption would come without penalty.

Adding a hymn to my prayer, I couldn't help but hum the Fanny Crosby tune I knew from childhood, "Rescue the Perishing." While much of the song is steeped in an evangelical fervor I don't much appreciate, I still found some wisdom in the third verse.

> Down in the human heart, crushed by the tempter,
> Feelings lie buried that grace can restore;
> Touched by a loving heart, wakened by kindness,
> Chords that were broken will vibrate once more.

Meanwhile, above my cabin, Becky and the guide sat in the ship's lounge, a bit bloodied by their efforts. The thorns were almost as bad for them as they'd been for the booby. Fortunately, there was another rescuer on board in the person of an emergency room physician from New York. He stitched their wounds with skin adhesive, and we were all, as they say, sailing happily into the sunset.

Finally, a travel warning: If you travel, your children may become infected with the travel bug. If they do, they may travel around the world and stay, thereby breaking your heart and making you proud.

Last year, my wife and I flew to San Pedro Sula, Honduras, to visit my daughter and to bring three suitcases of books donated by my readers for Honduran children. The visit inspired some spiritual perspective into the privileged life I live as a North American.

For instance, there's nothing like flying into the murder capital of the world to bring perspective to the biblical question: "For what is your life? It is even a vapor that appears for a little time and then vanishes away."

According to a 2014 UN Global Study, San Pedro Sula is the world's most dangerous city with three murders a day, making a Honduran life almost 15 times less valuable than anyone else's on the planet.

Those facts alone sent us speeding out of the city in our rented four-wheel drive and toward the rural town where our daughter, Sara, taught in a private bilingual school. Yet even at highway speed, we felt like we were passing from the proverbial frying pan and into the fire. Traffic accidents represent the second leading cause of violent death in Honduras.

Four hours later, we rolled into the darkened, foggy town of Marcala and checked in to our hotel.

Our work began early the next day when Sara introduced us to her fifth/sixth grade combination class at the Marcala Bilingual School. Soon we could see the education system offered another lesson in perspective.

The humble school was a well-kept two-story, cinder-block affair sitting atop a bare cement floor, protected from tropical rains by only a corrugated tin roof. Walls were well decorated while the windows were simple cut-outs in the cinderblock walls with steel bars to keep out the unwanted.

Sara assigned us to teach the English block, so each day we gave grammar lessons, graded papers, proctored exams and played charades with English vocabulary words.

The lessons inspired perspective into the difficulty of learning English as a second language, a language with 42 pronounceable sounds. The use of the definite article makes English particularly tricky. But, trickiest of all is that most verbs have three forms. Still, the kids persevere because they know that English brings increased opportunity.

We ended our lesson just before lunch so that we could distribute some of the donated books to Sara's class. We unzipped the suitcase and quickly witnessed a fresh perspective into the quenching power of books to a thirsty mind. After selecting small piles of books, the children returned to their desks where they read the books aloud to one another.

Thirty minutes later, we were eating our lunch and watching the kids play soccer when Sara pointed out a slight ninth-grade boy. "That's Jaime," she whispered. "He's a real math whiz. You should go meet him."

So I did.

During the next several minutes, Jaime inadvertently revealed some perspective into the privileges of being a North American versus a Central American.

Speaking in perfect English, this storeowners' son described the joys of playing video games and riding a bike. But most of all he enjoys studying. "I want to go to Harvard or Yale," he added with a naïve confidence.

When I reported back to his teacher, my daughter was moved by his determination.

"I hope so," she said. "Unfortunately, our town doesn't have a bilingual high school, so he may have to settle for public school where opportunities are limited."

Finally, when I think of all the things travel does for us, I think about the perspective it gives us into the life of the poor. This perspective is what Jesus was talking about when he said, "…to whom much is given, from him much will be required." (Luke 12:48).

After Sara's story ran in my column, many readers sent in generous donations to help Jaime. Those donations helped to inspire Sara to remain in Honduras where she now runs a nonprofit organization called Chispa Project. The project solicits book donations, inspires teacher development and sponsors international volunteer projects to Honduras.

On the project website, www.Chispaproject.org, Sara says the project gives direct ownership of the books to local schools and then trains the teachers and the PTA (padres de familia) to jointly manage the books. So far, donations have allowed her to send over 7,000 books to more than 40 different schools.

Please visit her site and see how she's done more than just survive in such a violent place, but she's learned to thrive! While you are on the site, consider helping these children learn. Consider it to be a travel trip of the heart.

4

BUILDING RESILIENT FINANCES

No, this isn't the chapter where I pull out the spreadsheets and send you to a financial planner, estate planner or tax planner. This is the place where we pause to consider what our finances bring to our life. Does money really buy everything you need? Or is there more?

Could you, would you, imagine a reality in which you had to live the lyrics from Lee Greenwood's "God Bless the U.S.A."? I mean what "If tomorrow all the things were gone I'd worked for all my life and I had to start again with just my children and my wife."

That was the haunting scenario I imagined in September of 1999 when Hurricane Floyd was cocked and loaded a few hundred miles off Cape Canaveral. In preparation for the blow, I began installing aluminum hurricane shutters over the house containing all our earthly belongings. With each screw I tightened, I felt like I would end up on the wrong end of that screw.

After the last shutter was installed I went back into the darkened shell and began selecting all the important stuff I needed to take. Then came a knock on my only un-shuttered door. It was my engineer friend from across the street stopping to make sure his neighbor had a place to go. He knew I was from California and earthquakes were much more to my liking.

Truth is, I was longing for a real good earthquake about then. Earthquakes aren't so bad. They are like putting all your stuff in a shake-and-bake bag. Your stuff gets messed up, but it remains in the bag. In a hurricane, your stuff blows into next week and one week starts to look like the next. Your neighbor's stuff is on your door and your stuff is in China. I'd prefer an earthquake where at least I can find my stuff. I might not recognize it as my stuff, but at least it'll be a pile comprised of just my stuff.

I told my friend about my preference for earthquakes, but he ignored me and transitioned into "engineer speak." He calculated the wind strength, elevation of beach highway and the elevation of our house. As he talked about the rising tide he delivered a serious conclusion with a joking smile.

"Don't worry," he said, holding his hand above his head and marking a spot against the wall, "the water will rise to about here. It won't flood your entire house."

After he left I went about trying to put my kids back together. They were going through their stuff, washing it with their tears, trying to figure out what was too important to lose. Truth is, I was doing the same thing. Things had seemed hopeful before my friend's visit. It seemed like we were doing all the right things to protect our stuff.

Jesus once had a visitor who also felt like he was doing everything right to protect his stuff. He had kept the laws of his religion and done all the right things since childhood, but he still lacked a spiritual center. He approached Jesus to ask him what must he do to become whole.

Jesus told him to obey the laws of his religion, but the man insisted that he had done all those things since childhood. Then, sensing that the man was still imprisoned, Jesus told him that there was still one thing he lacked – "go and sell all your 'stuff' and give the profit to the poor and your treasure will be in heaven."

The scripture tells us that he the man left sorrowful because he could not bear to lose his stuff – even if it meant saving his soul. "What does it profit a man," Jesus would later ask, "if he gains the whole world but loses his soul?"

If this rich young man could not decide what stuff was important, how was I going to decide in the face of this hurricane?

The next day, as the hurricane was spinning up to a category 4, my wife and I started the engines of our separate cars. Our evacuation plan involved her taking our four children to Becky's uncle's house in Orlando while I would report for duty at the military storm shelter for those who didn't have a place to go.

I followed my wife's car out of town and over the causeway evacuation route. I was still pondering whether I remembered to pack all the important stuff as we approached the intersection of our planned separation point.

That's where I saw it. The answer to my question of whether I'd remembered to take everything.

Pressed up against the back glass of my wife's station wagon were my four kids waving good-bye kisses.

"No worries," I thought as the tears welled, "I've remembered all the important stuff."

The lessons of that evacuation were in my mind in the spring of 2015 when I made a big financial announcement in my column.

"Next month, my wife and I will take a huge step. We are going homeless. But don't worry. I won't be on the street corner waving a sign, 'Will preach for food.'

"By homeless," I went on to explain, "I mean we'll no longer own a house or owe for it. By homeless, I mean "less of a home," downsized in a big way.

Yes, we've gone minimalist. We've sold our 2,800-square-foot home where we spent 13 years raising four kids, three dogs, two guinea pigs and one corn snake.

No more McMansions for us. We're renting a doublewide mobile home for the next year to help us transition into an itinerant retirement. We aren't taking any children or animals, only what will fill two bedrooms. The move slashed our living space by 1500 sq. ft. and our monthly housing budget by $1000.

If shedding that kind of material wealth is something you find unimaginable, you're in good company. The truth is that this level of sacrifice inspires us, but few of us actually do it. Don't get me wrong. I'm sacrificing very little. I've managed to sell my home and belongings at a fair price and will receive a sizable tax deduction for what I've given away. Most of what I've shed hasn't been used for years.

Nevertheless, our life change has made me take a hard look at the value I place on my stuff, especially the stuff I so drastically thought I needed, but never used. The whole event has me asking myself, when will a person feel satisfied that he has enough stuff or enough money?

The answer is — never. You'll never be sure you have enough.

The only thing you can really do is draw a bottom line on your net worth and determine that it will be enough. You must resolve, "This has to be enough. I will make this work. I will make it so."

To make such a decision requires some perspective. I found much of that perspective in 2005 in the devastating aftermath of Hurricane Katrina. That was the year I was temporarily deployed to New Orleans as the chaplain to the 1/179 Infantry Battalion, 45th Brigade of the Oklahoma Army National Guard.

I accompanied eight-man squads as we patrolled our sector of the steamy city. From the backseat of a Humvee, I saw folks watching us with uncertain eyes, unsure if they should thank us or blame us for not coming sooner. You could see the abandonment haunting those left behind, discarded and marginalized. Like something out of a zombie movie, they wandered abandoned roads searching for food and shelter.

Every patrol was a dirty, dangerous and often gruesome job carried out with the same seriousness of combat. We patrolled in full "battle rattle," the maximum amount of gear a soldier is expected to carry: helmet, goggles, flak vest, tac vest, pistol belt, canteen — essentially our "go to war" pack. Along side me was my chaplain assistant Sgt. Paul Jump, a 6-foot-4 member of the Osage Tribe carrying an M-4 rifle.

Our sector was a working-class neighborhood with shotgun homes sitting on elevated stilts or sloops. If no one answered our knock, we used our master key — a 20-pound sledgehammer. In each home, we looked for survivors, looters or bodies. We sometimes found all three.

The irony was that we came offering help, but we carried guns. Yet the guns were needed as we watched so many otherwise law-abiding people succumb to corruption. Looters broke open doors on blocks of stores using stolen cars and even a forklift to carry away more stuff. People used the storm to finish their quarrels. Criminals settled scores with police officers, and a few bad officers settled scores with whomever they pleased.

My most notable recollection is the odor coming from the rotting stuff of personal belongings. It was a hybrid of every possible sewer odor with every imaginable stink from the city dump. Floodwater sloshed through our doorless Humvee, baptizing our feet with gagging brown slush.

The entire experience reminded me of the words from the homeless Galilean man who declared in his Sermon on the Mount, "Don't store up for yourself treasures on Earth, where moth and rust destroy, and where thieves break in and steal. For where your treasure is, there your heart will be also."

You might say this was Jesus' version of the modern truism, "You can't take it with you," or "You'll never see a hearse pulling a U-Haul trailer."

In the meantime, I will admit that my newfound minimalism isn't a complete transformation. We both find ourselves holding on to all we possibly can. Does anyone know where I can rent a cheap storage unit?

If you think we're crazy, you're not alone. Our financial planner, who almost choked at the news, asked us why we'd made "such a whopping change."

It's a question I couldn't completely answer, but I tried to explain how we were preparing for an itinerant life of retirees. But spiritually, I knew it was more than that. Home ownership in the 'burbs seemed more and more about the obesity and audacity of materialism. We had filled every room and decorated every wall. It was time for a change.

We drew a line in the fiscal sand to declare that we had more than enough things. We said goodbye to all the stuff that weighed us down. We saw wisdom in the biblical admonition from Hebrews 12:1 to "throw off everything that hinders and the sin that so easily entangles."

So, on July 1, 2015, during Sacramento's record-setting 109-degree heat, we hired three men, two boys and a truck to squeeze the remains of our 2,800-square-feet of home furnishings into a U-Haul. We drove north out of our manicured subdivision and then literally across the proverbial tracks toward our new neighborhood. We followed the moving van in our cars and were soon caught up in a jam of older-model cars. Their drivers reflected the racially diverse community, which the 2010 U.S. census identified in 2010 as 70% non-white.

During our 15-minute convoy, the street noise intensified with delivery trucks and two passing freight trains. The social scenery changed drastically, too. Youths loitered outside a convenience store and shirtless men gathered in a liquor store parking lot. Crime here is 167% above the national average. I now have a 1 in 13 chance of becoming a crime victim.

Twenty minutes later, we arrived at the park, and I punched the gate code. Three other cars entered on my coattails. My sense of security faltered until I entered the park, where I found an island of well-kept homes.

The new neighborhood seemed quiet enough to be a golf course. The only noises I heard were Shar-Peis and poodles yapping through open porch doors as retired residents bid them to stop. Flags, wind chimes and bird feeders swayed from cleanly swept porches. A gaggle of geese crossed the road, a covey of quail scurried beneath the shrubs and a nest of rabbits scampered for their holes.

We passed over ten speed bumps before finally parking our truck in front of our new, yet old and very dated, mobile home. As we unloaded the contents, our movers expressed what we already knew – "This is very different," making the comparison with our old home.

"Different" was putting it mildly. We've transitioned from a privileged community to a modest, working-class community. There are no libraries, no golf courses or health food stores. The nearest Starbucks is five miles away, and the booms in the distant night aren't fireworks.

After the movers finished, my wife and I took a breather on our living room couch to look out our window into the shaded playground. We watched a dad play catch with his son, a retired couple strolled by while our neighbor unloaded his work truck.

My wife turned to me and said, "I feel at peace here."

"Me too, sweetie." I said. "I just hope our financial planner finds some of that peace."

Our idealistic resolve was tested just months after our move. For instance, we noticed that the home is a strong candidate for urban renewal. Unlike the surrounding homes wrapped with insulating wood, ours retains its original tin skin.

Our air conditioner runs nearly 24/7 trying to cool the tin box, and I fear our electric bill will double while cooling only half the space of our previous home. Large sections of the skirt are rusted over. Our thin plate windows are no match for the Sacramento heat — much less the barking Chihuahuas of my unemployed neighbors.

After three weeks of fruitless waiting for keyed access to our community pool, Mrs. Chaplain loses her cool. She slams the drooping and misaligned kitchen drawers and says, "These things don't work! And neither does the dishwasher. When is your friend going to fix this stuff?"

I thought he was "our" friend, but hey, I get the picture, so I relay her message to our landlord. Then I grab my "honey-do list" and head out our un-lockable back door on a mission to find the hardware to fix drawers, hang curtains and position pictures on our panel walls.

At the local Stuff-Mart, I browse the aisles, keenly aware that I'm no longer part of the home-owning haves. I'm now an official "have-not." I don't own a home, so I won't be buying much here. My landlord won't reimburse improvements, so it's not necessary to fill my cart with a dining room chandelier or a bas-relief garden fountain.

I return home where Becky and I start installing our non-reimbursable enhancements in the master bathroom. Becky's job is to line the rickety cabinet shelves with contact paper and then unbox a standing toilet-paper dispenser.

While she's busy with the paper-work, I step into the bathtub to install a new showerhead; I feel the thinning tub floor sink an inch beneath my feet. After finishing our repairs, I ask for privacy so I can initiate our toilet. A few minutes later, I frantically call for a plunger when the aging porcelain coughs up brown debris.

To cite an over-quoted Oz-ism – we really aren't in Kansas anymore. We've crossed the proverbial tracks. I fully realize this the next morning when I chirp my car lock twice and startle a homeless man camping a few parking spots away.

I can't help but think how the bearded young man resembles Sunday school depictions of Jesus as a homeless man healing the sick and helping the poor. A comparison Jesus himself made when he self-identified as "... the son of man who has no place to lay his head."

We aren't homeless; we're only house-less. We live among the poor, but we aren't even close to being poor. We can easily buy our way back into the suburbs. And maybe we will, but for now we will settle down for the journey, write about it, and strive to live content with what we have.

I started a new job as hospice chaplain along about the same time we settled in the mobile home. In that job, I crisscross nearly 1,000 square miles of Sacramento County to visit terminal patients in their homes. The conversations can be heavy, but in the chatter of my initial visit, someone invariably asks where I live.

Lately, I've noticed that it's harder to answer that question.

By "harder" I don't mean that I'm getting early onset of "old-timer's disease." I can certainly remember where I live. By "harder" I mean embarrassing.

It's embarrassing because we've traded our subdivision life of manicured lawns, jogging paths and backyard barbecues for a 40-year-old double-wide mobile home on the less-desirable south side of Sacramento.

The first time I fielded the question, I answered evasively, "just Sacramento." I worked the subterfuge because I knew that if I 'fessed up with "South Sacramento," I'd see the person's demeanor change into something that implied, "Shouldn't your education and income level put you into a nicer neighborhood?"

Even when I finally did reveal my hidden location, I'd feel it necessary to include a full narrative describing my intentions to simplify and downsize. I guess that was my way of saying, "I'm not poor. I'm just pretending to be poor, kind of like an embedded reporter."

If my confession makes you want to send me a nastygram or leave me a fuming voicemail, you wouldn't be alone. Said one incensed reader of my downsizing: "You have a choice where you live. If you really want to know what poor feels like, give away your profits." The reader was channeling Jesus' teaching that it was "easier for a camel to go through the eye of a needle than for someone who is rich to enter the kingdom of God."

I get it. I really do. My feelings are a convoluted concoction of hypocrisy, but my feelings are also complicated. They're complicated by the fact that while my modest digs embarrass me, I'm also ashamed of being ashamed. I'm ashamed of my need to explain that I'm not poor, while adding the qualifier that I'm not really rich.

My feelings are also complicated because, like most Americans, I consider myself a common man. Like many of you, there's one thing I'm ashamed of more than being poor — I'm ashamed of appearing rich. Yet, we are rich. By world standards, if you enjoy regular meals in a climate-controlled home with a car in the garage, then you're rich. Few of us are "common." We are, in fact, highly privileged. Third World citizens appreciate little difference between the average American and one of its most famous citizens, Bill Gates.

"Why don't you just move back to the subdivision?" you may ask. Good question.

For now, I think it's apparent that God needs a little more time to teach me the Buddhist-like advice first dispensed in Philippians 4:11-14 by that fire-breathing prosecutor, the Apostle Paul. While recorded in many translations, I think the modern paraphrase of "The Message" befits my goal here.

"Actually, I don't have a sense of needing anything personally. I've learned by now to be quite content whatever my circumstances. I'm just as happy with little as with much, with much as with little. I've found the recipe for being happy whether full or hungry, hands full or hands empty. Whatever I have, wherever I am, I can make it through anything in the One who makes me who I am."

Paul learned that it's much more important how one lives his life than where one lives his life. Of course he learned that lesson from living many years in a prison. Let's hope my learning doesn't take me that far.

My motive for moving has been questioned by several of my readers. While some thought our modest move was admirable, most questioned the sanity of trading a manicured subdivision for a manufactured home surrounded by industrial parks.

However, one reader in particular — let's call her "Mrs. Chaplain" — thought my columns overstated the downside of our downsizing. Normally Becky's my best editing voice, so I listened to her insistence that I write a retraction for exaggerating the negatives and understating the positives.

I told her it was hard to see those positive attributes during my morning fitness routine that crosses a dangerously busy street to join a running path along the southern side of an electronics plant. As I round the backside of their compound, I turn north along the railroad track where homeless folks rise from their camps in overgrown fields and from beneath creek bridges. Nevertheless, she thinks that I should emphasize the upside of our downsizing. For instance, she likes the quiet surroundings and the wildlife of birds and rabbits.

When I complain of how I sometimes miss our cavernous two-story house, she pushes back.

"You don't miss our house. You miss our neighbors."

She's right.

We miss our old cul-de-sac. We miss the fix-it advice we got from Melvin and the good food we got from Thomas and Lupe. I even miss sharing Neighborhood Watch stories with Michelle, the nurse across the street. I don't really miss Mike's practical jokes but I could use more of Les' golf tips.

Gratefully, we're staying in touch with old friends, but we're also making new ones. My young neighbor, Taylor, built a gate for me to keep my yapper dog inside our patio. My other neighbor, Joe, attends church with me and also drives me to the airport for my speaking engagements.

"So," you ask, "how are you are doing with your downsize?"

I think we're doing well. That's because we took with us those things that make our house into Norris and Becky's home. We brought our beds, our art, our favorite chairs, our family photos, golf clubs and holiday decorations.

But, more important than furniture and mementos, we brought a sense of ourselves into our new home. We brought our adventurous spirit, our consciousness of togetherness and an understanding of what is essential in life. We brought our faith.

Maybe that's what Proverbs 24:3-4 means: "By wisdom a house is built, and by understanding it is established; by knowledge the rooms are filled with all precious and pleasant riches."

Hopefully, that answers the questions from my readers and hopefully Mrs. Chaplain won't think I downplayed the downside of downsizing. Couldn't resist that one.

Financially, the move has been a bit confusing, especially in our church life. Lately it's felt like our senior pastor was giving me the stink eye. Problem is, I couldn't figure out why or what I was feeling. It took a month, but I finally realized why I was getting the stink eye. I'd accidentally stopped making my monthly church donations. My oversight occurred in January after I enrolled in our church's online contribution system.

My mistake happened as I was setting up the initial test payment on my credit card. If it worked well, I'd start making semi-monthly debits and rack up frequent flyer miles. However, when making the initial payments, I forgot to add more. The result was I hadn't given so much as a penny in four months!

As a Protestant, I don't normally confess to my pastor nor does he track my giving. However, since some congregants express their unhappiness by withholding contributions, I thought I should set the record straight with him. Of course I was too much of a coward to tell him directly, so I went to our administrative pastor instead. (Kind of like picking which parent you'll least disappoint.)

"Norris, I'm so glad you mentioned it," he said. "Our bookkeepers had asked me if you were upset with us."

"No, no," I insisted. "We've been quite happy here for 12 years. Please forgive my senior moment."

"I can understand that," he said. "Most of us check our credit cards and bank statements looking for fishy charges and to see if somebody took something from us that they shouldn't."

"But," he added, "most of us fail to stop and count what we should have given, but didn't."

He was right.

There were no fraudulent charges in my monthly statements, so I had focused only on my healthy bank balance. I hadn't bothered to ask why the balance was higher than normal. I took the spend-now-audit-later approach. I was looking out for No. 1, thinking about getting what I deserved — never mind what I ought to be giving to those in need.

Instead of limiting my search to fraudulent charges, I should have been looking for the places I'd failed to be generous. I should have been looking to see if I shorted someone, not just if someone shorted me.

Jesus told a story in Luke 12:13-21 about a greedy farmer who produced such a terrific crop that he asked himself: "What can I do? My barn isn't big enough for this harvest."

His answered himself by tearing down his barns to build bigger ones. Then he sat back and said: "Self, you've done well! You've got it made and can now retire. Take it easy, and have the time of your life!'

But the next night, the dude died and stood before God to answer this question– "Fool! Who gets your barn full of goods now?"

Jesus concluded with a warning: "That's what happens when you fill your barn with Self and not with God."

After confessing to my pastor and promising to right my wrong, I felt better.

The administrative pastor had only one request.

"I think your story makes a good point. Can I share it with the congregation? Anonymously, of course."

I agreed because, while Protestants might do confession, this was a good opportunity to do public penance for such a boneheaded mistake. In the end, the pastor wasn't giving me the stink eye nor was he monitoring my contributions, but after he reads this, he probably should.

Fortunately, getting my tithing straight also helps me some during my annual meeting with my tax accountant.

"Your stories always make me cry," my tax accountant told me last month as she calculated the tax liability I'd assumed by selling our house and moving into a rental.

"Yeah, well," I said stammering at her early estimations of my taxes owed, "It looks like it's going to be my turn to cry today."

Taxes often make us cry. And it was no different 15 years ago when a young church member approached me asking for help with his taxes. Phil was a new member who was demonstrating a leadership many found inspiring. I was happy to help him.

As he positioned his pencil over our worksheet, I began asking the typical interview questions. In moments, we'd found our way to the most discouraging part of his financial picture. Phil made good money, but had paid very little taxes during the previous year.

I told him he shouldn't worry; after all, he owned a home and had child-care expenses. But my comforting words would prove premature.

"OK, how about your child-care costs?" I asked.

He threw out what seemed to be an indiscriminate estimate.

"OK," I said, enunciating my reply, as I knew his mother-in-law did the family child care. "You paid the kids' grandmother that much?"

"No, but isn't that about what most people pay?" he asked.

"Phil, the IRS doesn't work that way." I explained that his claim needed to be the actual dollars he had paid.

Nevertheless, he penciled in a number.

"How about contributions?"

He shrugged and volunteered a figure of about $100 a week. Again, I knew we were talking rough estimates.

"So," I said, "You should have the receipts from the church?"

He shrugged again explaining that he'd always thrown cash in the collection plate, never bothering to record the amount on an offering envelope. He assured me he didn't contribute for tax purposes — only for God.

As he penciled in yet another estimate, I had a sinking feeling his boat had sprung a big leak in some deep waters.

We have a saying in the hospital: "If you didn't chart it, you didn't do it." The saying embodies the idea we can claim integrity in our job, but at the end of the day, integrity still seeks definition and measurement.

Phil claimed integrity in the strongest of voices. But his protest was one of entitlement. Phil was certain that everyone — including the IRS — should trust him just because he said so. By refusing to allow his integrity to be measured, he was risking being labeled the thing he most detested: a cheat.

Each year, thousands of us — even people of faith — give way to the temptation of naming their own figures and not just on our tax forms. Yet, the temptation isn't really so much about dollars as it is about placing ourselves in authority.

I recalled an old story about a woman who is offered $1,000 for illicit relations with a rich playboy. When the woman agrees too quickly, he stammers trying to adjust his price.

"Er, uh, I meant $100?" he countered.

"Absolutely not! What kind of woman do you think I am?"

"Well," he said, "I thought we'd already established what kind of woman you are and we'd gone to haggling over the price."

When I left that day, Phil was still haggling with his integrity. I'm not sure what he ever decided to put on his return. But whatever it was, I can't help but wonder whether he would ever discover there just aren't any deductions for being a person of integrity, only additions.

Finally, charity must be the basis of all our financial priorities. It's one well expressed in the wisdom of 13th century Rabbi Moses Maimonides who wrote the "Eight Degrees of Charity. His list is a great way of assessing our charitable abilities. I propose we end this chapter by counting down Maimonides' priority list and see where you place in these charitable motives.

8. Giving unwillingly. This is the least of charitable actions. Tibetan Buddhist Trungpa Rinpoche called this kind of giving, "idiot compassion." The problem is that we're only giving because we don't want to feel uncomfortable for our own wealth.

7. Giving cheerfully but giving too little. This happens when we drop a dollar in the Salvation Army kettle. We smile generously, but we know a buck is woefully inadequate.

6. Giving only when asked. This can be a large or small gift, but no matter the amount, we give only because we're pressured to give.

5. Giving without being asked. This giving comes about during our search for a genuine need. It's depicted in the old Kaiser Cement Corp slogan — "Find a need and fill it."

4. Giving to those we don't know, while making sure they know who we are. We make sure the recipient knows who we are perhaps

because we need them to be indebted to us. Confession time — I find it hard to go higher than this one.

3. Anonymously giving to someone you know. Perhaps you give your pastor $200 to buy clothes for the Jones' family and whisper, "Don't tell them who gave this gift." It's a high form of giving, because it concentrates on the need and doesn't solicit applause.

2. Mutual anonymity — Neither the donor or recipient know of each other. This is hard because there's simply no payback for you at all — no building with your name on it, no gratitude and no tax deduction.

1. Giving your time or money to help someone become self-reliant. This is best illustrated in the saying, "Give a person a fish and he eats for a day. Teach him to fish and he eats for a lifetime." It's extremely difficult, because your gift is really you.

This type of giving is the radical kind Jesus introduced in Mark 12 after he observed a poverty-stricken widow giving all she had in the form of two coins worth half a cent.

""Truly I tell you, this poor widow has put more into the treasury than all the others. They all gave out of their wealth; but she, out of her poverty, put in everything—all she had to live on."

While most of us haven't topped Maimonides's sage list, I wonder what would happen if we'd aim for at least the fifth level where we give without being asked.

It's simple enough. Start by going to the website www.charitywatch. org where you can pick a legitimate charity and contribute something before the charity has to spend the money to ask you.

I can't be sure, but if Maimonides were alive today, I suspect that's what he'd do.

5

FINDING RESILIENCE IN FAMILY

These days the word family has a lot of different meanings, but to the general population it almost always involves marriage and children in some form or another. While there will be more changes to the family structure, I believe we will always have marriage and children.

Therefore this chapter isn't so much about how to have a happy marriage or raise happy children. Those methods and secrets change over the years. Besides, if I knew the secrets, then you'd be paying good money for this book and I'd be a fairly rich chaplain. No, this chapter isn't a how-to-succeed chapter as much as it is an attempt to share the stories I've seen. As you read them, I hope you find a bit of yourself and unlock some of the answers you need.

First, let's talk about the weddings. As a minister, I officiate dozens of picturesque weddings with all the pageantry of limos, gowns and tuxedos. During these ceremonies, I stand before a couple as they publicly proclaim poetic promises accompanied by an elegantly performed love song.

It's easy to see the exchange of wedding vows as the most beautiful part of the ceremony, but as a chaplain who's been doing this marrying-burying thing for more than 30 years, I'll tell you that nothing matches the beauty of watching those vows when they are being fulfilled by someone who meant what they said when they promised, "For better or for worse… 'til death do us part."

To this day, I've never heard a love song as beautiful as the serenade that came from the room of a 45-year-old cancer patient in 1991. That was the year I was doing a one-year chaplain internship at Medical Center.

The song drew me down the hallway toward the room where several staff members were gathering outside the door. Inside the room, lay a jaundiced patient with a liver that was clearly failing. All of his organs were failing; doctors were measuring his life in days, if not hours.

So, into his bed came his wife Anne of 22 years, and maybe all of 98 pounds. She nuzzled alongside him, stroking his face, as he strummed a John Denver medley. After about 10 minutes, he switched chords and nodded toward his eavesdroppers as if to ready us for his finale.

His wife took her cue by sitting up in bed with crossed legs, brushing her hair behind her ears and wiping her tears. Then she stared deeply into his dark eyes as if going toward a preplanned rendezvous with his soul. She clearly knew what was coming. For it was her song, "Annie's Song."

"Come let me love you, let me give my life to you," he began with a crackling voice. He stopped for an unwritten rest beat, forced a smile and pushed farther into what seemed a prayer set to music.

Let me drown in your laughter / Let me die in your arms

Let me lay down beside you / Let me always be with you

Come let me love you / Come love me again

While a few of the staff members held their professional composure through the songs, it's a safe bet that our stoicism didn't last through the entreating lyrics, "Let me die in your arms."

The physical and spiritual intertwining I witnessed in this couple sharing a hospital bed will always recall for me the scripture from Genesis that says, "This is now bone of my bones and flesh of my flesh…."

It's a wonderful moment when couples pledge their togetherness with "until death do us part," but it was a sacred moment to behold this couple turn their "I do" vows into a goal-line declaration of "We did." Brother, that's love. Sister, that's pageantry!

In the opening month of the eighties decade, my wife and I said, "I do." And by the grace of God and our love for each other, we will bring this love well into the 21st century.

Truthfully, most ministers would rather do a funeral than a wedding. My wife didn't want me to tell you that. She says the preference sound morbid, but she knows that there are at least two reasons for the partiality.

First, the minister's personality isn't always suited for the pageantry details of a wedding. On the opposite end, clergy will often do exceptionally well with the personal pastoral care required at a funeral.

Second, wedding participants are very particular about details; funeral participants have simple requirements, such as good empathy and a caring presence. That's not too hard for most pastors. But, at a wedding, if I so much as mispronounce a middle name, my name is mud.

For those reasons, planning starts with premarital counseling. The first question often is about the honorarium. Because of a few memorable moments I've had in the past, I require payment in advance.

Two incidents inspired this requirement. Once, a groom stopped our march toward the altar, exclaiming, "Wait!" He then extended a $100 dollar bill toward my face, saying, "Here ya go, Bud!"

Another time, a bride summoned me to her dressing room, where she met me in the doorway in her slip and push-up bra. She positioned her checkbook on the doorjamb and insisted I accept her check that instant.

During our premarital session, I always try to clarify a few rules. One year after rousing a drunken groom at his home wedding, I added the rule, "No alcohol before the wedding." One "smart" couple brought their keg to the church parking lot — presumably to drink after the wedding.

There have been times when I've declined to marry a couple. For instance, one young lieutenant whose wedding I was going to officiate came to me a few months before the wedding. He said his fiancé was uncomfortable with that "whole death thing." She wanted him to ask me if it would be a "deal-breaker" if they left out the till-death-do-us-part concept. Yup. I assured them it would be.

One of my most memorable deal-breaking moments came in 1995 while I was serving as an active duty Air Force chaplain in the San Francisco Bay Area. I got a call from an active duty helicopter pilot asked me point blank, "Do you perform *all* weddings?" I told him yes, but he put an odd emphasis on the word "all," that I thought I should qualify my answer.

"I'm a Protestant chaplain and I do *all* Protestant weddings," I said. I'm not sure he heard my limitations because he still scheduled the pre-marital counseling.

The couple came to my office that afternoon holding hands and in good spirits. After a few minutes, they asked to see a written copy of the ceremony I would use.

They were studying the script together when the pilot blurted out a question. "Would it be possible for you not to talk so much about God?"

When I offered them both a blank stare, the woman added some explanation. "Our friends are going to be offended if you mention God and the Bible."

I wanted to ask if they noticed the cross I was wearing above my left uniform pocket. Instead, I tried to gently explain that I couldn't officiate a Christian wedding without using Christian vows because I was, well, a Christian.

At that point, the woman leaned forward in her chair and made her confession. "I should have told you — I'm Wiccan."

"Yeah," I said, "You definitely should have mentioned that."

Don't get me wrong. As a group, Wiccans are generally peaceful and tolerant people. They are a nature-based religion. They do have witches, but not witches in the sense of potions and spells. They don't worship the devil, in fact they don't believe in the devil.

"I can't do the wedding," I said, "but perhaps you can get a Justice of the Peace."

The woman nodded in agreement, but I could see that her fiancé was getting furious.

"But you said you did all weddings — no matter what denomination," protested the pilot. At this point, you need to understand that military members are entitled to use the chapel with no charge and chaplains aren't allowed to charge for their services. The result is that we get a lot of calls from bargain hunters who have never been in church. And this pilot was one of them.

I reminded him of our phone call when I said I do Protestant weddings and I tried to explain that Wiccans aren't just another break in the Baptist church. The pilot remained unmoved.

The woman confronted her fiancé with a question: "Dear, don't you understand? We would be hypocrites for saying the Christian vows and the chaplain would be a hypocrite for officiating a wedding for people he knows don't believe the Christian vows."

Wow, I was under her spell. Her words were so profound that I have repeated them to nearly every engaged couple who has come to my office.

This Wiccan had a sense of her own worth, but her fiancé was more interested in bargain hunting for a free wedding – to the point of denying something that was important about who she was. He was a bargain hunter trying to smuggle God into a relationship where God was not wanted. And the truth is that God only comes to marriages as an invited guest.

We often try to haggle the price of our integrity. We try to hide who we are because showing who we really are might cost us something, but in the end, if we have to conceal who we are, if we sell out who we are, it has cost us everything.

Finally, my funniest wedding story took place a few weeks after my own wedding when I got a phone call from our photographer. He asked that Becky and I return the church in the upcoming week wearing our full wedding regalia. Apparently every single picture the photographer took of us as a couple failed to develop. Becky and I were forced to re-enact our ceremony. Gratefully as we approach four decades of love, I think our marriage continues to *develop* quite nicely.

Marriage is a risky proposal at best. But few weddings I've done in the past 30 years were as fraught with risk as the one I performed a few years ago in the acute unit of our local VA hospital.

It all began when a nurse sent me to a room reserved for our more seriously ill patients. Inside, I introduced myself to a man in his 50s, small in stature and weak in the face. Sitting beside him, a woman held his hand under the bedcover.

"Your nurse tells me you want to get married," I said.

The couple locked their starry eyes and nodded in affirmation.

"When?" I asked.

"Now," they said.

"I don't know if that's..."

"Don't worry, chaplain," the woman said. "I've researched it online. I know it can be done."

"Well, I'm not sure..."

"Chaplain," the groom interrupted. "I'm dying."

I paused to consider my answer, not so much from the spiritual side, but from what our risk management department would say. They'd probably ask if the couple was in love or if the woman was just after the patient's pension.

Even if their intentions were sincere, risk management would never allow it if doctors thought the patient's pain medication affected decision-making capacity.

"Why now?" I said in a thinly disguised way of asking, "Why have you waited until now?"

"We've planned it several times during the past two years, but his lung cancer delayed all attempts," she said. They'd even managed to get a wedding license once before, but it expired when medical appointments and family drama interrupted.

"We're tired of delays. Today seems like the right time," she said.

The woman outlined a step-by-step process of the requirements. First, we'd need a doctor's notarized signature. Then she and I had to go to the county clerk's office for the license. After that, we'd return for the hospital ceremony, then circle back to the clerk's office to finalize it all.

The paperwork was easy enough to accomplish on our end. The doctors signed off, so the risk management department had no objection. However, the woman lacked transportation to the clerk's office.

"I'll take you," I said, even though I knew our risk management folks would have a coronary if they knew I was transporting a family member in my personal car.

But I did it anyway.

By late afternoon, I finally stood before the couple. The bedridden groom wore a rose on his chest. The bride managed to freshen her look with a little makeup and a discounted bouquet from the hospital gift shop. A dozen hospital staff members stood witness.

A few minutes into the ceremony, I asked the couple to repeat after me their promise to stay together "in sickness and in health...'til death do us part."

Without hesitation, they echoed the traditional vows. Suddenly, there wasn't a dry eye in the house.

Promising one's love is always risky and this couple knew that truth better than most. They knew what sickness and health meant — and within a few months she'd discover what it meant to be parted by death.

At the end of the day, they'd stood "before God and this company" to declare their eternal love with his literal dying breath. And for me, as it turned out, I avoided the biggest risk of all — the risk that comes from not doing the right thing.

The only secret I know about marriage is the one I normally share during the wedding ceremony. I've shared that secret with many couples as I officiate weddings in backyards, churches, forests and living rooms. I begin those ceremonies by saying, "If you were to ask me what is the most important lesson I've learned in my almost 30 years of marriage, I'd have to tell you that love is a choice, not a feeling."

I don't ask the couple about their love. I know they love each other. Attesting to love is only a testimony of the present. Instead I ask them to make radical promises of their future will. That's a much scarier proposition.

I ask them to make willing promises about loving, comforting, protecting and forsaking all others. Will they be faithful? Not until love parts, but rather, as long as they both shall live?

"I will," they both declare.

I once was approached by a couple with handwritten vows that declared their promise to stay married until "love do us part." I politely asked them to find another officiator, because this chaplain always will say, "till death do us part."

Eighteen months later, the love she had for another man parted the newlyweds.

Why didn't this marriage last? Why do so many fail? I wish I knew the complete answer to that question, however, I believe it often is because people don't realize that wedding vows are everyday, not just on the wedding day.

If taken seriously, the future promise of the will means that they look for ways to perform acts of kindness and compassion, whether practical things like doing their fair share of housework, or relational things like good listening.

In my house, this is the kind of willing love that keeps on going whether I burn the toast or burn my temper. It is the kind of love that tells me I am forgiven before I can ask. It is the kind of love that "halves a sorrow and doubles a joy."

Like many couples, my wife and I sometimes go to bed dead tired. We easily can find ourselves too tired for the fun I seek and too tired for the cuddling she requests. But we rarely are too tired to talk out our day and absolutely never too tired for our three good night kisses and "I love you."

It's the intentional building of a relationship where independence is equal, dependence is mutual and our obligation is reciprocal. This kind of daily choice — day in and day out — brings something deeper and far more lasting. It brings Jesus' words to pass, "The two shall become one flesh." (Matthew 19:5)

Without a daily commitment of the will, relationships easily degrade. It's too easy to become like the husband who stopped telling his wife he loved her. She confronted him with this deficiency and the husband replied, "I told you 'I love you' on our wedding day. If I change my mind, I'll let you know."

That husband was sorely confused. The bride was right. We have to declare our love on a regular basis. But most importantly, we also have to assert our will to make things work — till death do us part.

Sharing a bed is also another secret of marriage. My wife and I have managed some difficult sleeping arrangements over the years. At times, we have slept in beds that aren't much bigger or any more comfortable than a hospital bed. Other times, we have determinedly pushed two single beds together.

Our determination to share a bed reminds me of a time that a nurse sent me into a room to visit with a couple who'd shared a cramped bed their entire marriage. Sadly, the husband had just passed away. The room was filled with family pictures and mementos that intentionally communicated to the staff that this man was not to be identified by a room number or diagnosis. He had a name, a life and a family that loved him.

The bed swallowed the frame of this slight man enough to allow his wife to perch on the edge in the top corner of the mattress. She leaned into his stiff, sagging shoulder and held his hand while caressing his arm. His eyes were closed and his mouth open.

As I sat and talked with the family, the wife told me she had shared a bed with this man for 58 years. During all of that time, the couple had only a double bed — not a queen or king — just a double bed. Now she was wondering how cold the night would get without him.

"I just can't understand it," she said. "So many of our friends buy these big beds. They say they need the room. The beds are so big, you lose each other."

She told me there was always enough room in their bed, because from the moment they slid in, both had their emotional compass set for a life-long commitment. In the center of the bed, they found each other's hand and, so entwined, peaceful sleep came easily.

Now, in front of us that afternoon, a permanent peace also had come easily. He was resting, and, at her advanced age, she was likely to join him soon in a place where their souls would permanently entwine.

As I looked at this couple, it occurred to me that I often am witness to the pageantry of many formal and elegant weddings, but the beauty I witnessed in this room was rare. This was the final fulfillment of the vows, "for better or for worse, 'til death do us part."

The marriage that began with this vow had now seen fulfillment in this bed. Through the years, I have heard a lot of reasons for breaking those vows. Perhaps Jesus hit the nail on the head when he explained that Moses had been forced to approve the breaking of marital vows because of "hardness of hearts."

Somehow, I think this couple discovered hard hearts are softened in smaller beds. That's a lesson that I hope I will always remember as our bed continues to be our nightly meeting place for years to come.

Mary and Joseph didn't have much of a bed at all. If you've read the Christmas story, you'll know they managed with just the hay in the barn. And if you read the story in detail, you'll know that it was a miracle in itself that their marriage began at all.

For you see, if this was a Christmas gossip column in biblical times, I might title it, "Test results show Joseph not the father; parents of alleged Savior considering divorce."

Yes, embedded in the Christmas story is a line from Mathew 1:19 not usually emphasized in candlelit church readings. "Joseph, her (Mary) husband, was a righteous man and did not want to expose her to public disgrace; he had in mind to divorce her quietly."

As a chaplain I'm often asked the difficult question: What does God think of divorce?

I wish I were asked easier ones like, "What does your wife of nearly 28 years think of divorce?" While I might facetiously reply, "That depends on the hour of the day she's asked," I'd likely recount the plan my wife spelled out long before our wedding: "Never joke about divorce and never threaten it. Don't even plant that seed of thought."

Good plan.

In the beginning, God had some plans, too.

Nearly 28 years after Jesus' teenage mother escaped a likely stoning, he risked a similar fate by recounting God's plan to some religious leaders who were asking what God thought of divorce.

Jesus quoted the original specs for the human race in saying, "God created this organic union of the two sexes (and) no one should desecrate his art by cutting them apart."

These leaders challenged Jesus by noting that Moses' teachings allowed for divorce. "Moses provided for divorce as a concession to your hard heartedness," Jesus retorted, "but it is not part of God's original plan."

The key words here: "as a concession to your hard heartedness." Divorce isn't a part of creation, but because we all experience a hardening of our hearts, divorce can happen.

"Hard heartedness" is a way of describing resentments. Maybe these resentments took place during the marriage, or long before you met your partner.

These resentments cause infidelity and all relationships will break under the weight of infidelity. However, don't be too quick to settle with the sexual definition of infidelity. I think God's definition is much bigger than that.

Infidelity happens when one or both people stop working the vows, not just the vows to be sexually true, but the vows to be truthful, the vows to work with each other throughout difficulties and the vows to share each other's hurts.

When one or both people stop working these vows, divorce will most often be the result. So what happens then? I think it pays to remember two things.

First of all, God feels the hurts from all broken relationships. God hurts with our strained relationships at work as well as our strained relationships with countries like Iran. God hurts when he sees broken relationships with children as well as weakening relationships in our places of worship.

Seeing God as one who hurts with us gives us more perspective, because instead of seeing us as locked in our own battle of hurts, we realize we are also hurting an innocent party. We are hurting the one who has created us to live in loving relationships.

I think this perspective gives me energy to do my best to heal those relationships, whether they be at work, home or in world politics.

Second, and most important, God works with us to heal relationships. The healing may take place in our current relationship or it may take place while we are inside another relationship, but healing will always be God's business.

After all, when I see what God did through the scandalous birth of a child named Jesus, I become more and more convinced that restoring and healing relationships is what God has always been about.

Not all relationships can be healed. Take Tiger Woods, for instance. Just after the Associated Press named him Athlete of the Decade, he might have easily been labeled Addict of the Decade. Woods was leading a double life with doubled troubles.

Multiple adulterous affairs in such a short marriage are more common to the acts of a sex addict than they are of your common adulterer. People who misbehave at this level aren't merely guilty of off course antics as described by the press; this is an addictive behavior.

While late-night TV had their fun with Tiger jokes, sexual addiction is no laughing matter. Like all addictions, it strikes people in all walks of life, from the skid-row pervert to the office manager.

It even strikes people of faith who do their best to follow the admonition of their faith. For Christians, it's found in Galatians: "But among you there must not be even a hint of sexual immorality . . . because these are improper for God's holy people."

Most of what I've learned about this subject, I've learned from the counseling of "God's holy people." As a chaplain, I've heard spouses promise before God that this would be their last time. I've heard them weep until they thought they'd squeezed every last ounce of sin from their soul, only to see the addiction return.

This especially is true for the sex addict whose mainline is Internet pornography. I've sat with spouses who've wept over their fears of inadequacy to their husband.

"Haven't I offered him enough?" asked one especially beautiful wife.

"You absolutely have," I assured her, "but this whole thing isn't about sex. It's not about you. It's about his addiction."

What makes this addiction particularly problematic is that there is no public support for the sex addict as there is for people who are addicted to food, alcohol, drugs or gambling. Most employers or family members will react in supportive ways when these addicts seek treatment.

So, forced into secret, sex addicts take the only way they know. They try the white knuckle or cold turkey cures. They apply all their willpower because they have to keep making a living. They lie to themselves promising that they will change. "This will be my last time!" they swear. But, alas, it's not.

Thankfully, there are serious treatment solutions for this addiction. The treatment road starts with an assessment test. The Sexual Addiction Screening Test was created by the foremost expert on the subject, Dr. Patrick Carnes, to assist in the assessment of sexually compulsive behavior. You can find it at Carnes Web site, www.sexhelp.com.

If you have the addiction, however, treatment cannot begin without acknowledging the common adage: "Admitting you have a problem is the first step to recovery."

That's why the most common treatment successes are found in self-help groups like Sexaholics Anonymous (sa.org) or Sex Addicts Anonymous (sexaa.org). Both groups practice the basic principles of recovery found in the Twelve Steps and Twelve Traditions of Alcoholics Anonymous. Furthermore, many churches sponsor Celebrate Recovery groups. Find your local group on the internet.

Woods truly is a legendary golfer, but can you imagine how truly great he can be with treatment? Can you imagine how much better you can be? Get help. Get it today.

When The Two Become Three

Often, the love between two people will bring about children. While marriage is an act of love, having children becomes an act of faith. By choosing to have children, parents are choosing, by an act of faith, to love them no matter what. That love was lived out most eloquently between the parents of Jesus, Mary and Joseph.

Unfortunately the Bible doesn't give us a detailed journal of their parenting, but I can imagine what it was like for them in the early months. In my mind's eye, I can see them waking early one morning with the crowing of the roosters.

Their boy awakens, pawing at the air and fussing for a feeding.

Mary opens her robe, offering her son the fullness of her morning milk. Mother and son hold the moment as theirs while Joseph finds renewed sleep.

Soon, the sun streaks through the barn's crevices, flooding it with light and Mary with questions she can no longer contain.

"Joseph."

He groans.

"Joseph."

"What is it, Mary?" he asks.

"Tell me again what the angels said."

Joseph rolls over and props himself on his elbow.

"The angels said, 'Don't be afraid.' "

"But, Joseph! How can we not be afraid? We're so young. We have nothing."

Joseph rubs his eyes, hoping to find the clarity befitting Jesus' stepfather.

"I'm not sure," he says. "But maybe 'nothing' is what we're supposed to start with. After all, God made an entire world from nothing."

When Mary offers only a respectful nod, Joseph drops his head.

"You're right to be worried. I'm worried too," he says. "How will I provide for you both?"

Mary reaches for Joseph's face, cradling it with a warm hand. "I love you," she says.

It is Mary's answer to most of Joe's worries.

Joseph's fingers trace Jesus' hand as a means to answer his own question.

"This hand will carry a hammer," Joseph says. He then stretches his hands apart as if to bracket the sign he envisions. "We will be, 'Joseph and Son Galilean Carpenter Shop.' "

"According to your angelic friends," Mary counters, "these hands will also carry 'great joy!' "

Mary moves Jesus to her other side and invites Joseph to entwine himself with them.

"Will he change the world?"

"I'm not sure the world is ready for him," Joseph says.

"They won't be, but this is God's timing. Not ours."

Mary counts Jesus' toes aloud, contemplating how to categorize him — man or God — when she dares a deeper question.

"What if God should want to take him back?" she asks.

The loss of his firstborn seems unimaginable, even if it were somehow God's will. Joseph does his best to deflect his fear through a question of his own.

"There's only one thing that really bothers me, Mary. Who are we? How did we get so lucky?"

Mary stares at the thatched roof in contemplative silence. She is absorbing that word 'lucky' when Joseph revises his question.

"Or should I ask, 'How did we become burdened?' "

"Joe! Watch what you say!"

"But, honestly, who are we to be trusted with such a great task?" he asks.

"We are nobody." She pauses a few moments before adding, "Or, maybe we've been chosen because we are everybody."

"That makes no sense," he claims.

"Yes, it does. Everyone will have to decide what to do with Jesus — just as we did."

He remained unimpressed.

"I'm not sure I can fully answer your question except to say, mankind is a part of God's plan. I'd even say we are his plan."

At that, Joseph shakes his head. "Goodness. Do you suppose God has a plan B?"

Mary puts the sleeping Jesus aside and rightly answers Joseph by playfully stuffing his shirt with a handful of straw.

"I love you," she says, "but I have one more question."

"What?" he asks.

"Can we please get some more sleep while we still can?"

Sleep was the only thing on my mind at 3.a.m. when I answered the call from the Labor and Delivery Unit of Sutter Children's Hospital.

"Chaplain, we have a baby not doing well," the nurse reported. "Her parents are asking that you 'please come.'"

Thirty minutes later, I stood at the mother's bedside listening to her tell me of her journey through a problem pregnancy. She'd nursed thin hopes that doctors would find things to be more fixable than previously predicted. But now it was obvious that the baby had underdeveloped lungs and a leaky heart, and mom was wrestling with the doctor's recommendation for birthday surgery.

"Had God just teased us?" she wondered. "What do we have to do? How do we pray? Would it help to baptize the baby? Can you baptize her? We've got to do something! She's got to have a chance."

In my Southern Baptist tradition, we don't baptize babies. But those who would argue theology at a time like that have never looked into the eyes of desperate parents and heard them plead, "Do something, Chaplain!"

So, I asked the nurse to help me wheel the mother into our Neonatal Intensive Care Unit where we could have a prayer.

Pronounced "nick-you," the unit is a world of wires, IV bottles and backlit beds. It's very close quarters, where doctors, nurses and respiratory therapists squeeze through tangled tubes to deliver highly specialized health care to the tiniest people you'll ever see. But as cramped as it was, the staff made room for us when we arrived for this "emergency blessing."

I opened a bottle of sterile water and placed a drop on the baby's forehead. My prayer was simple: "Hold this child in your hand and help her hear your voice. Bless his life, in the name of the Father, Son and Holy Spirit."

With that, Momma's whimpers melted into weeping as she took her daughter's tiny hand and — finding a spot that wasn't wrapped, poked or monitored — she placed a kiss in that tiny palm and whispered something into those tiny fingers. Then, as if she had placed a thing of priceless value in her daughter's grip for safekeeping, she closed it tight.

This mother's love reminds me of the miraculous way God whispers his love into the hand of each of us when we are born — placing there a promise that, no matter what, he will never let us go. And having pledged that love to us from our first breath to our last, he wraps our fingers around that promise for safekeeping.

The Apostle Paul wrote "For I am persuaded that neither death, nor life, nor angels, nor principalities, nor powers, nor things present, nor things to come, nor height, nor depth, nor any other creature, shall be able to separate us from the love of God, which is in Christ Jesus our Lord."

I sometimes forget how personal and deep God's love is for each of us. As a minister I often talk about the depth of God's love, but it took witnessing this mother's heartfelt whisper into a tiny hand to remind me that God's love is forever present.

I'll never know the exact words that she entrusted to her daughter's grip. But in the coming weeks of miraculous procedures and risky surgeries, the real miracle was that this child never released the grip of her mother's promise — and three months after her birth, she went home a healthy little girl.

Miracles were common occurrence in our Neonatal ICU. Take for instance, Miguel and Bahar Torrente. Bahar was a 32-year-old Iranian-born Muslim. Miguel was a 41-year-old Colombian born Catholic. Both were public high school teachers, and Miguel serves his adopted country as a helicopter pilot in the California Army National Guard.

They were married in a Catholic ceremony followed by Muslim vows at the reception. Two years later, they had a healthy child named Bianca.

In the spring, Bahar returned to labor and delivery for the birth of their second child, but doctors sent her home saying it was false labor.

Bahar repeated that scenario the next day. On the third day, Bahar was insistent, it was the right day — in more ways than one. Arianna was born normal, but six hours later, worried about the baby's color, Bahar consulted a nurse who immediately began giving oxygen.

Unknown to the staff of this small hospital, Arianna had something called pulmonary atresia. The American Heart Institute Web site defines this as a "condition in which no pulmonary valve exists. Consequently, blood can't flow from the right ventricle into the pulmonary artery and on to the lungs."

Simply put, Arianna's heart had no capability of pumping blood back to her lungs, so oxygen was useless and Arianna was dying. But on this day — the right day — there walked into the nursery a visiting doctor from our hospital. The only doctor on site qualified to make the diagnosis; Dr. Andrew Juris ordered a steroid given that would buy precious time.

As the staff readied her for transport to Sutter Memorial in Sacramento, a priest baptized Arianna and family members prayed over rosaries, medallions, Bibles and Korans. "This was interfaith," as Miguel recalls, "friends of all faiths and churches were praying."

When Miguel and Bahar arrived in Sacramento, pediatric heart surgeon Dr. Richard Mainwaring met them. The doctor explained Arianna's condition and the series of surgeries he would perform in repairing her heart.

The Torrentes were feeling like things were coming together as some kind of divine plan.

But before Bahar would consent to surgery, she insisted a chaplain be called for prayer.

I arrived in our NICU holding no prayer book specific for Muslim/ Catholic families. So, I simply began praying the Lord's Prayer. As I prayed, both families were reverently respectful. Then I pulled out a Muslim prayer and softly asked permission to read it, too.

Both families nodded and after I read the prayer, I could see in their tears that both prayers had found their marks in listening hearts. It was a faith that gathered the hopes of a mother with the intentions of our creator and molded into something much more powerful than the prayers of one.

"This was the hardest thing we've gone through," Miguel admitted to me by phone this week, "and it can make or break a relationship, but this made it stronger.

"Having had Bianca, we were grateful, but you can't imagine how grateful until you have (a) sick child."

"How is Arianna right now?" I asked.

"Oh boy," the pilot said. "Other than a scar, she's a wild child!"

Well, Arianna may be a wild child, but after all that, I think we can definitely say she's God's child.

Neonatal ICU stories could be sad too. A few years later, I answered another phone call. This one came from our nursing supervisor.

At first, it seemed she was calling with a typical request. "We have some parents asking for you to bless their newborn daughter," she said.

"No problem," I answered.

"Actually," she said, "It could be a problem. This child is dead."

I was quiet for a moment while the supervisor pushed more information. The baby had been born on Christmas Eve. Now, instead of wrapping the babe in swaddling clothes, the parents were shopping for burial clothes.

"I can," I promised.

"Good," she said, "But you'll be alone."

"Pardon me?" I asked.

The nurse unwrapped a bit more of the story. The parents had left the hospital immediately after the death, too devastated to remain. Nevertheless, they wanted the baby blessed in their absence.

"No problem," I said.

A few minutes later, I met the supervisor in the basement morgue. The busy nurse pointed to the refrigerator that sheltered the baby and then returned to our short-staffed ICU.

Alone, I opened the refrigerated space to see a bundle wrapped in blankets with a nametag attached. I checked the tag. Yes, I had the right baby.

I picked up the little girl and began removing the safety pins that kept her so tightly wrapped. I wanted to see her face.

I peeled away three layers of blankets until finally I saw her ashen face peeking through the covers. Something about the experience felt like uncovering a lost treasure embedded in a sandy surface.

That's the moment, I realized that maybe I did have a problem: How could I pronounce a blessing if no one was present to hear it? It felt much like the old adage — if a tree falls in a forest and no one is around to hear it, does it make a sound?

According to most religious practices and beliefs, the baby was already in heaven. There was nothing I could do to speed her journey or even obtain better accommodations. Knowing all these things in my theological brain was very different from knowing these things with the heart of a parent.

Then, against all the classroom theology I'd ever been taught, I decided to speak from my heart.

"Hello, sweetheart," I said. "You were someone's promise — someone's anticipation and expectation. Your mama and daddy love you very much. I know because they asked me to come and tell you that one more time."

After "talking" to the baby, I pronounced a blessing and prayer for the parents:

"God, I entrust to your care this life conceived in love. May your blessing come upon these parents. Remove all anxiety from their minds and strengthen this love so that they may have peace in their hearts and home."

I rewrapped the baby and gently placed her back onto the refrigerated shelf.

Had this been a real blessing? I wondered. Would the parents be able to know, to feel, to hear the blessing? Or had this just been the proverbial tree falling in a forest?

Within my heart, I knew something had happened, but what? Then I realized that blessings aren't always about what someone does for another. Sometimes they can be what happens to the one doing the ministry.

On that day, it felt like both.

One of the biggest blessings in our married life came just before Christmas in 1989 with the visit of a social worker to our home.

I say blessing despite the fact I often joke with people telling them to never let social workers in your house at Christmas time. I say that because it was my experience that social workers can be like the Wise Men of the nativity story bringing unexpected news.

I jest about this, because it was during Advent of 1989 that social worker Richard Costa came to our house with news of great joy about our adoption application. Over Christmas cookies and apple cider, Richard got to the point.

He told us he'd found a 3-year-old girl who would fit well with Sara, our 5-year-old birth daughter.

"Her name is Brittney," he said, "and she comes with some conditions."

We could hear the gears turning. While there seemed to be a light at the end of this two-year tunnel of adoption requirements, we couldn't help but wonder if these unforeseen conditions might be the lights of an oncoming train.

First, Richard said the foster family, who had kept this child for the past 15 months, wanted updates and an occasional visit.

Maybe we were just eager, but that seemed to us a reasonable request.

"No problem," we said.

"Second," Richard breathed before telling us the girl had a baby brother named Michael who was recently added to the same foster family.

"If you take the girl," he said, "you must be willing to consider the boy if he comes up for adoption next year."

Shaking my head, wondering how I would provide for a growing family on a clergy salary, I suggested we take the holidays to think about this.

The truth is, I guess I was looking for some kind of sign that this was supposed to be it. Was it too much to ask for a star and some wise men?

My wife didn't need to think about it. She immediately started looking through Sara's toys and things for anything that might be unisex.

Was there a baby blanket in a closet somewhere with a little more blue than pink? Surely all the inflatable bath-time baby books could be used for a boy and a girl.

Four weeks later, we went to the foster home for a visit. I think we were all interviewing each other when, feeling the nervous need to impress the foster parents, I asked, "Did Richard tell you that I'm a minister?"

"He didn't have to," replied Aurel Gion, the foster mother, "That's what we prayed for."

This was it. This was our sign. And it was a helpful sign to us when, three years later, we were adding Brittney and Michael's unexpected sibling, Nicole.

Since then, not a Christmas has gone by in which I've not thought of that sign. For, like the social workers, the Magi of the Nativity also looked for a sign.

"And this will be the sign to you," the angel said to Wise Men. "You will find a Babe wrapped in swaddling cloths, lying in a manger."

Does God always give you a sign for such life-changing events? No, not always, but I am praying that this chapter becomes a sign for a select few of you to consider the adoption option. Maybe it's time to invite a social worker to your home for Christmas cookies.

Adopted kids aren't always grateful though. You'd think that choosing a child through adoption would instill them with a great sense of gratitude that they were saved from a rough life. Yes, you would think, but you'd be wrong. They will still live their lives with the recklessness that youth imbues. A few years ago I was 400 miles from home, teaching a military marriage class in San Diego, when my bedside phone rang at 4 a.m.

The first words I really heard was, "Dad, she stopped breathing!"

My son was referring to the same daughter who had recently recovered from sudden and unexplainable multiple organ failure.

He went on to explain that he and his friends had been pushing their disabled truck on a dark country road when another car rear-ended them. The boys jumped clear of the car, but my daughter wasn't so lucky. Her brother found her in the driver's seat, slumped over the steering wheel, convulsing.

"But don't worry," he said, still in the voice of the former Marine, "I saved her with CPR." He assured me that she was now breathing, talking and vomiting.

Now it was my turn to breathe.

"Dad! Are you there?"

"Yes. Oh, my God, yes. I'm here."

"The paramedics just put her in the ambulance," he added. "Mom is on her way."

And so was I. Two hours later, while waiting for my return flight, I called for an update and learned that my daughter was getting a CT scan. The good news was that my daughter was talking, but it was what she was saying that I found troubling.

"God must want me dead," she told my wife in a sardonic reference to her second brush with death in 30 days.

The 90-minute plane ride home gave me pause to think where her remark fit into her life. Our lives intersected 18 years ago when I opened an envelope that contained pictures of a blond-haired, blue-eyed, 2-year-old girl. The pictures that spilled onto our kitchen table were from the people who had fostered our first two adopted children. The letter was an unofficial notification that our children had a sister.

"Looks like we're going to have another child," I told my wife.

"How can we do that?" she asked, the type of question asked after an accidental pregnancy.

We were already struggling with many of the difficult issues faced by blended families. How could we find the patience for this many children? Neither our car nor our military quarters seemed big enough. How could our hearts possibly be big enough?

Within the next year, we returned to her foster home. It was during that visit that our hearts were captured. God had a plan for this one to join her biological siblings and became facetiously known to her new parents as "Little Bit."

Six hours after receiving my son's phone call, I was "wheels down" on the runway of my home airport in Sacramento. When flight attendants allowed phone calls, I got more breathtaking news.

"She's being discharged," my wife told me. "Just a mild concussion." She then instructed me to come to the house where my wife predicted I'd find them all asleep.

As I drove my car out of long-term parking and onto the freeway, I kept thinking about my daughter's sardonic conclusion that God wanted her dead. But having had a front row seat to her early years as well as her recent brushes with death, I remained convinced that God does have a plan for her.

With that in mind, I sang my rebuttal all the way home — "Au contraire ma belle fille. On the contrary, my beautiful daughter. Very much, au contraire."

I'm grateful my children made it into adulthood, but sometimes I find myself missing those early days when they thought their parents were omniscient. When they were young, we did all we could to promote the mystique that my wife and I were all-knowing. My wife warned them against hiding things from her because she had eyes in the back of her head.

One day, my wife was working on a puzzle with our daughter when our son, Michael, decided to test her assertion. Coming up behind Becky, he worked his preschool hands through her recent haircut until he got his fingers on her scalp.

"Michael! What are you doing?" she asked.

"I'm looking for the eyes in the back of your head."

Michael's oldest sister, Sara, laughed because, even at 8 years old, she knew that her mother had only one set of eyeballs. However, later that night, Sara tested her own theory as to the source of her mother's wisdom by taking scissors into the bathtub where she tried to copy her mother's latest haircut.

When my wife came to retrieve Sara from the tub, she found hair clinging to scissors hidden among bathtub toys. It was definitely a middle name moment.

"Sara Elizabeth! You cut your hair!" Becky exclaimed.

Sara, shocked that her mom noticed what she'd considered subtle cuts, erupted in tears asking, "Did God tell you?"

"God tells mothers many things," she said. "Right now, God is telling me to put you to bed early."

I, too, grew up thinking that my mom was sagacious. Whenever I had a question, I asked it until my propensity for random interrogatives finally earned me the unflattering family nickname of "Question Box."

By the time I was approaching puberty, my potential to ask embarrassing questions grew exponentially. I suppose it was my mother's attempt to suppress these awkward queries that caused her to enroll me in the junior high's sex education program.

Unfortunately for my mom, every question answered in Mr. Bolivar's sex education class spawned a dozen more. I had nowhere to bring my curiosity but to Mom.

One night while Mom drove my brother and me home from Royal Ambassadors, (RAs is the Southern Baptist version of Boy Scouts,) I popped off a question I'd been holding for days.

"Mom, do women really get pregnant every time they have sex?"

"I don't know," she said as blankly as though she was considering the possibility of rain.

Thinking my inquiry needed mathematical clarification, I added, "Well, since you only have three kids, you must have had sex with dad only three times. Right?"

She didn't answer. She just drove. The fall air created an awkwardly silent veil that reminded me of the time I'd asked my Sunday school teacher if God could create a rock he couldn't lift. Maybe I finally asked my mother the unanswerable question.

Mom drove in a distracted silence for another half mile until a bright railroad-crossing signal lit the night air. Mom slammed the brakes and brought us to a halt just over the safety line. A thumping on the car roof told us that the crossing arm was trying to hold us in place.

Panicked, my mom mashed the accelerator as she said, "Norris, quit asking so many silly questions."

I looked out our back window. The sight of a splintered crossing arm swinging like a broken metronome at the oncoming train brought to mind the Bible verse we'd learned in RAs.

"Children, obey your parents … so that you may enjoy long life on the earth."

The irony did not escape me that I was almost killed asking about sex before I was old enough to enjoy it.

"Yes ma'am." I said and stopped asking her so many questions.

My father was a bit different from my mom in that he always welcomed our questions. He was a Baptist fundamentalist who loved people more than a fight. However, when battles were waged on behalf of his parishioners or friends, he could be a fierce fighter.

I was 11 years old when he took the opportunity to reinforce just how much people mattered to him. My lesson began on a summer vacation day at our community pool where I was swimming with my 13-year-old neighbor, Jerry.

At some point, Jerry began asking me to distract bikini-clad swimmers so he could get a submerged close-up of their anatomy. I refused to be his co-conspirator, so I called him a pervert and left the pool in protest.

He followed me to offer his comment — a punch across my jaw. I answered with a single blow to the backside of his hard head. We separated to opposite sides, like boxers nursing our wounds.

At home, my father found me in the kitchen icing my broken hand. When I told him my story, he surprised me by with a slight criticism. He was disappointed that I hadn't used his oft-repeated advice to plant a tight-squared fist on the nose of my opponent.

Then he pulled back the kitchen curtains to look toward Jerry's house. He thought he'd seen early promise in Jerry, but now sounded unsure. "Jerry needs to know that people aren't objects for his selfish use," he said. "Hopefully, you helped him see that."

I didn't really understand my father's commentaries until a few weeks later when he was interviewing for a pastor's job in a Southern Baptist church. His "interview" consisted of preaching a trial sermon, meeting with deacons, and eating a family dinner with an influential member.

After church, I felt underarm stains forming on my newly dry-cleaned suit while we drove to our host home. When our hostess greeted us at her front door, she offered to store our purses and suit coats in a hall closet.

I declined her offer, retracting my plaster cast deeply into my bulging sleeve.

A boiling pot summoned our hostess back into her kitchen, so my father took the moment to question my behavior on such a warm day.

I knew that these dinners were more about interviewing our family for a good fit into the church, so I explained that I was trying to hide my cast.

Why?" he asked.

"They won't want to hire a pastor whose son gets in fights," I said.

At that point, my father dropped to his knees to meet my flushed face and nervous eyes.

"You won't embarrass me, son," he said. "Family is more important. In fact," he added with a hand sweep of our surroundings, "you are more important than all this." Then he simply stood and began removing my coat, like a ringside trainer freeing a fighter's robe from quivering shoulders.

My father's lesson that people are more worthwhile than personal gain, job advancement or poolside popularity remains a difficult lesson for me to live even today. However, I find strength in his example of loving people where they are, how they are, and because they are God's children.

The church didn't hire my father, but at the end of the day, my dad and I knew that we had won the fight.

In other matters, dad could be quirky. For instance, his favorite bible verse was "Abstain from all appearance of evil." (1 Thessalonians 5:22) The verse is a catchall for those who condemn what the Bible doesn't specifically oppose.

In my father's case, it was alcohol. No surprise given the fact that our church covenant asked members "to abstain from the sale and use of intoxicating drinks." The only problem we found was in teaching Jesus' water-into-wine miracle. The wine was purportedly "the most excellent grape juice."

My dad was so obsessed about appearance that our cars were banned from the local liquor store that also doubled as our small town convenience store. After all, he reasoned, a bag filled with milk and bread might be imagined by the town gossip as restocking our secret liquor cabinet.

To make matters worse, a Catholic family in town owned a van identical to our uniquely two-toned Dodge. When people asked my dad how our van came to be seen at the local bar and, of all things, Saturday night Mass, he humorously, but adamantly, claimed a case of mistaken identity. These inquisitors must have missed the line in our church covenant urging members to "avoid all gossip, backbiting and excessive anger."

Still the questions continued right up to the day my dad backed into another car while exiting his parking space. Fortunately sobriety brought a divine inspiration. He took the van to a body shop where it came out in three new tones — a true reversal of colors.

His teachings were well ingrained in me when I was hired by Thrifty Drug as a clerk in my hometown's first strip mall. When I told the manager that I couldn't sell alcohol from my checkout stand, he apprized me that prohibition hadn't been regionally reinstated. No sale, no job.

As few parents would be, my parents were proud of my new unemployment. So, when the new Safeway opened next door to Thrifty Drug, our family went on a shopping spree. Overwhelmed by variety, each of us packed the cart with our choice of cereals, but when my dad tried to write a check for the whopping $100 total, the checker directed him to the manager standing behind the liquor counter for check approval.

Inspired by my Thrifty stand, my father announced that he'd not be seen at the liquor counter, while the manager kept his post in front of a wall of brown bottles. It was a contest of the wills and the loser was the poor clerk who had to restock our groceries while my father marched his empty-handed family from the store.

Given this upbringing, I was 19 before my Baylor roommate dared me to guzzle a beer. I hated the taste of it … both coming, and a few seconds later, going. Ten years later I joined the Air Force reserves, where my priest colleagues taught me to enjoy a good wine.

I have few complaints that my father steered his children from alcohol. However, I suppose if I find some sadness around religious teaching, it's when it becomes too focused on what we are supposed to abstain from, rather than what we are supposed to be drawn toward.

Over the years I've found more value in verses that teach positive action, like Psalm 34:14: "do good; seek peace and pursue it." I suppose that means if you're looking for good, you don't have time for evil.

Instilling faith in children isn't simple. When I recall my father's teachings, I must say he did very well with his efforts to instill faith in us. However, like many of you, I sometimes wonder if I could have done a better job instilling faith in my children.

It's a concern one of my colleagues shared with me one evening on a cross-country flight.

"Do your children go to church with you every week?" she asked.

"Yes," I answered rather flatly.

"Mine won't go," she said gazing through the darkened window. "If they do go, it becomes a fight and I end up crying through mass."

"Well, I have a few that give me some tears as well," I admitted rather slowly.

"They won't go?"

"Two go easily and the other two need some coaching, but getting them to go is the easy part," I admitted to her astonishment. "We've taken our children to church their whole lives, so they know as long as they are in our home, they will always go."

"Tough love, heh?"

"No, not really. It's kind of like seatbelts."

"Huh?"

"They never liked seatbelts when they were young but they learned the car doesn't move without seatbelts."

"My children go," I said pausing with an accent, "but that doesn't mean that they want to be there or that their faith is refreshed in the same way I experience."

"So, they're not resentful about not having a choice?" she asked, her voice conveying the suspicion that my children would spend their grown-up years in therapy. "I'm not sure giving them a choice is always wise.

There's a Bible verse that says 'Start a child in the way he should go, and when he is old he will not turn from it.' I think that suggests we are to give our children a faith tradition that may one day serve as a jump start and help them better understand the sincerity of their parents' beliefs."

"So you're admitting, 'You can lead a horse to water, but you can't make him drink'?" she asked

"You might say that. They may not choose to drink from spiritual waters, but we do have an obligation to be sure they are close to the well.

"I'm not sure how parents justify giving choices about something as deep as spiritual education when they don't give them choices about learning to read and write."

"But in the end," she stated, "We can no more choose faith for our children than I can fly this plane."

"Exactly, because the hardest part is still going to be how you live between worship services during the week. If you're not careful the message can get lost in the noise of church and I think children are especially tuned in to the hypocrisy factor."

"So, if our lives don't emulate the basic goodness we're are trying to demonstrate and maintain each week, then requiring our kids to go church every week won't help them live a life in which service to a greater good is a daily part of their existence. And I think it may be that last part that matters the most."

The plane ride and the discussion ended that night as most do – safely and without any new solution to world problems.

Bringing your children to church is a good start, but it's not enough by itself. We need to talk with them and explain why we go to church and thereby give them a glimpse into our souls.

Leading a good life where service to others is paramount does a great deal. We want our children to become the best people they can and we want them to be driven by more than habit. Children do not need to clone our faith, but in the end, parents need to be present with their child in their search for the meaning of faith and model that faith so that it can become the most potent and creative force in their developing life.

Despite all our efforts, our children definitely haven't cloned my faith. In fact I still remember once when my son said, "I'm not even sure there is a God."

It was about the most hurtful thing a child could say to a chaplain dad.

The questioning reminded me of two patients I'd met during my rounds as a pediatric chaplain. Both patients were pastors' children.

The first child was a 10-year-old boy with cancer. He lay in his bed, using controllers to throw punches at the villains in his video game.

He gave me a cursory glance to see whether I was medical staff bringing needles or anything else that might hurt him. I had no such instruments, just a harmless Dalmatian marionette.

He shot me a dismissive look that referred me to his father standing at bedside. I took my cue and turned toward his pastor dad.

"My guess is that you're finding a place for prayer during this illness?" I said, leading the conversation.

"Yes," the father answered, while stroking the head of his distracted son.

We spoke a few more minutes about the support faith brings to illness until a phone call took him out of the room.

Left alone with the patient, I asked him the same question about prayer that I'd asked his father.

For the first time, he took a long gaze away from the video, over his shoulder and past me toward where his father was engaged with his phone call.

Making sure his answer would be confidential; he silently shook his head.

"Not at night or when you're scared?" I pressed.

He did a double take toward his father and repeated his negative gesture.

A minute later, his father returned, and we cordially finished our visit.

Ready for some grown-up conversation, I caged my Dalmatian and went to see a woman with a high-risk pregnancy.

Upon realizing I was a chaplain, the woman discarded the common salutations to announce, "My father is a pastor."

No pleasantries. No, How-do-you-do?

I inferred from her tone that her spiritual needs were met in her DNA. Her dad was her holy guy.

Responding in a half-mischievous tone, I said, "Oh, really? We're both PKs (pastor's kids). Can I have a seat?"

She studied me and decided it might be OK to talk.

As we spoke, it quickly became apparent her dad was not her holy guy. In fact, her new spirituality was such a radical change from her Evangelical home that I was sure her dad now saw her as a member of a cult.

But what's a parent do to do when your child no longer sees any wisdom in your faith?

There really are only two things you can do. First, accept that we cannot choose our child's spiritual DNA. We can no more choose faith for our children than we can chose their love.

Second, take comfort in your own faith journey and recall the path God laid out for you. In doing so, your confidence will be renewed that God also will lay out a journey for your child, just as he did for you.

It's hard, of course. It means letting go in far deeper ways than just letting your child drive off to college. You have to let go at your core.

Letting go doesn't mean you approve of the route your child has taken, it simply means that you trust your child to the heavenly parent who gave you this child in the first place.

Inevitably, children want a pet. I suppose it's their effort to take on the parenting roles. In my family, I'm the "dog person."

My wife Becky loves animals, but she tends to reserve her respect for those that don't come into our house, such as humming birds and elephants, whales and eagles.

Given her lack of enthusiasm for dogs, I'm always grateful when she assumes the caretaker role for my pound pup during my cross-country speaking trips.

I'm careful to call Becky the "caretaker" because it would be a pitiful mistake to reference her as Toby's mommy. She will not share the "mommy" title with any sentient being except our children. You might say that stopping people from referencing their pets as children has become her "pet" peeve.

I think that's because she understands that our pet relationships are fairly straightforward compared to those with our children. If you give your pet affection and food, you'll definitely become its best friend.

Children are much more complicated. Having children is an act of faith. Parents can never know for sure if their child will become a rock star or a drug addict. A new parent can only wonder – will this child grow to love me or spend his or her life totally disrespecting me?

Abraham knew a lot about the uncertainty of parenting. He's the father of a boy named Isaac in an oft-told story from the Judeo-Christian tradition. This father-and-son pair went skipping up the mountain on a father-son camping trip. But all was not what it seemed. Abe was on a bizarre mission from God.

God told Abe to slay his son on that mountain as a peculiar way of proving his faithfulness. At first glance, the story seems like the tale of a god with a borderline personality disorder — pleased one moment and homicidal the next.

But at second look, we see God has a plan. Just as Abraham ties his son to the altar of sacrifice, a clueless ram wonders into the picture. Fortunately, God instructs Abraham to free his son in exchange for the ram.

Slaying one's son is the most unthinkable thing I can imagine. How can you look at your own flesh and blood and be prepared to kill something made in your own image?

Yet somehow, I think that was a lesson that God was teaching Abe. The father must first kill or relinquish the image of himself that he'd projected onto Isaac. Isaac needed to be freed of his father's ideals before he could become the person God created him to be.

In other words, Abraham walked out of faith. He had to let go of his son, give him up and let God shape Isaac's life. Abe had to trust that God alone could create an image of the holy in Isaac's soul.

I once knew a kid who folks said looked a lot like his father. Yet he continued to disappoint his father every time he came home with poor grades or was suspended for fighting at school.

So the father relinquished the image he had for his son and released his care back to God. His son was allowed to make several more mistakes, but they were his mistakes, and they led him on his own faith journey.

And guess what? Once my dad let go, I think I turned out OK.

However, to my wife's dismay, I did keep the part of my father's image that loved dogs.

6

FAITH – THE MOST POWERFUL F-WORD ON EARTH

The most important element of resiliency has to be Faith. It is the most powerful F-word on the planet, because Jesus promised that if we only had faith the size of a mustard seed, we could move mountains with it.

Jesus made the promise to his disciples after they asked him why they couldn't do the amazing miracles he performed.

Jesus' response is recorded this way in The Message paraphrase of the Bible: "Because you're not yet taking *God* seriously. The simple truth is that if you had a mere kernel of faith, a poppy seed, say, you would tell this mountain, 'Move!' and it would move. There is nothing you wouldn't be able to tackle."

That verse says a great deal about thriving and resilience. It means our faith is the key to overcoming and bouncing back from what's hit us in life. In my work in the hospital, someone is always telling families that if they only have enough faith, their loved one will survive.

Well, that's Hollywood faith. That's the kind of faith that performs tricks and magic. That's not the kind of faith I'm talking about here. I'm talking about a faith that has four major elements to it – Worship, Gratitude, Prayer, and Afterlife.

I start with worship because for many people this is the birthplace of their faith. Yet church is often the thing that hangs up people in their faith journey. I think that's because we sometimes invest too much magical thinking in the church. It's not a place of magic. It has what you bring to it. It's a rendezvous point to meet God, but it isn't where God lives, like a genie in a bottle.

So, if you're one of those people who've been hung up or even strung up by the church, I invite you to take a deep breath, as we darken the door of the church once again.

First, let me ask you a straight-up question. Why don't you go to church anymore? Can you explain it without tears? Or without anger? Was it the pastor who hurt or angered you?

During my more than twenty years of preaching, I can recall at least three people who threatened to drop out of my church or chapel if I didn't change my leadership. When I didn't change, they pulled their membership and promised they wouldn't be back.

The first person was a retired pastor who was upset with the time-saving method I employed for communion. My plan called for our ushers to pass the communion cups down one row while passing the wafer tray down the other row. They would then reverse the process until everyone was served.

The pastor emeritus saw the process as confusing for his aging wife, so he promised me that if I ever served communion that way again, he'd never return.

You guessed it. I did, so he didn't.

The second person was a member of the California Air Force chapel where I served. He came to me one day telling me that he didn't like me preaching about tithing in a government-sponsored chapel filled with retired congregants. (Tithing is the Christian teaching that encourages parishioners to give 10 percent of their income to Christian charities or churches.)

It didn't matter to the man that our chapel used the tithes for educational material and gave the rest to charity. He promised that if I ever repeated my preaching mistake, he'd never return to the chapel

Of course, I did and of course he didn't.

The third person was a young mother who had trouble with me illustrating my sermons with many of the sad stories I've written for this column. She told me that if I kept telling the stories, she wasn't coming back to chapel.

By now you must see the pattern in my stubbornness. I did and she didn't.

It's not unusual for parishioners to disagree with their spiritual leader. The Bible has several examples of it, but most especially in the pesky disciple named Peter.

When the authorities came to arrest Jesus, his disciple Peter drew his sword and slashed off the ear of one of the arresting soldiers. He was a loyal parishioner, but like my congregants, he definitely had his own ideas on how things ought to be run. The problem was that Peter's plan was in direct contradiction to Jesus' plan.

Now, I don't mention this story to compare myself to Jesus. I cite it because it shows how inevitable it is for people to get sideways with their faith community. I don't find fault with these people because it's in our nature to seek more fertile spiritual ground when things become uncertain.

Nevertheless, it's good to remember that a faith community should be a place where people are allowed to practice their faith. "Practice" being the operative word here. We won't always get it right, but nothing should keep us from trying.

"But it's hard," you say. I know it is. But Christian faith teaches that we need only to find a faith that is equivalent to the minuscule size of a mustard seed. Once we have that faith we can move mountains.

I'm glad I can report to you that my three congregants were grounded enough in their faith to avoid becoming spiritual dropouts. They found a new faith community and presumably a more pliable preacher.

Now if I can just find a more pliable congregation – or in my case, a more pliable readership – it would be a perfect world.

But again, probably not.

"How do I find a church?" asked an audience member at a one of my speeches. "I'm so disappointed with my previous attempts." Her question reminded me of an experience I had as a Baylor University ministerial student facing the same dilemma.

"Where are you going?" I asked my college roommate, Terry, as he readied to leave our pew in the middle of a sermon about the Church of Thessalonica.

"I need to find a relevant church where I can invite my friends," he said in a voice loud enough to awaken those not sharing our new pastor's interest in ancient cities.

With that, Terry bolted from the pew with his red-faced roommate chasing behind him. After all, he had the car. If you are like Terry and have bolted from your share of spiritual communities, let me recommend three qualities to look for in a church, synagogue, mosque or other place.

Look for a place that will reach up, reach in and reach out.

While those titles were popularized by the book "The Passionate Church: The Art Of Life-Changing Discipleship" by Mike Breen and Walt Kallestad, the concepts have been around since the early church.

Reaching up means we initiate a conscious contact with God. This is worship. I consider things like music, Communion and prayer as up-reach. This is the place most people talk about a heavenly feeling. If we place too much emphasis on up-reach, however, we become like the old saying, "Too heavenly minded, and no earthly good."

Reaching in involves the strengthening of relationships between the members. Some churches do this through small groups or religious education. These groups come together for regular study of devotional material related to their tradition's religious book. When a church spends too much time on reaching in, they become cliquish, egotistical and self-absorbed.

Reaching out means the church helps those outside their walls: spiritually, socially, financially and medically. My home church gives 10 percent of its income to the community. Once my pastor even gave away "spiritual stimulus money" to the parishioners and asked them to reinvest it in the community.

In my opinion, many churches have a dismal record in outreach. In an effort to compete with the business world, they have expensive buildings and high salaries and there is little left to give to those less fortunate.

Reaching out must, of course, be balanced or the church might as well become the Red Cross.

Good outreach is how a church grows and gets better at its mission. As I studied church growth in seminary, I was surprised to learn that most people come to church, not because they love their leader, the music or the pretty building. More than 70 percent come because a friend or neighbor reached out and invited them.

Wow, this is exactly what Terry told me about wanting a church where he was proud to invite his friends. Like me, he wanted a place where his friends could hear a message with life-changing potential.

Where did Terry take me that night?

We squealed out of the church parking lot in his Chevy Nova. We drove as far out of academia as we could get and turned into the gravel parking lot of a Baptist church in a little Texas town called Lacy Lakeview.

It was there we were relieved to find a church that was willing to reach up to a God of grace, reach in to teach God's forgiveness and reach out with love toward all.

Remember the better points of your childhood faith is the thing I often tell people who are struggling with their former spiritual traditions. I encourage them to look back and reconsider what was right about your childhood church experience, not so much what was wrong about it.

Perhaps that's what I was doing when my wife and I flew to Charleston, South Carolina, to visit our grandchildren, and also ended up revisiting the Southern Baptist customs of our childhood.

Our revisit began at the First Baptist Church of nearby Walterboro, where my daughter lived. Inside the church vestibule, a smiling usher greeted us with a bulletin. Like the mimeographed programs of my boyhood, the Walterboro missive told of the upcoming Vacation Bible School and listed the parishioners with June birthdays.

Once inside the sanctuary, I looked up at the vaulted ceiling, and I admired the way the stained glass diffused the morning light onto row upon row of burgundy-cushioned pews. I cast an envious look at the pulpit large enough to double as a confession booth, if Baptists were so inclined.

Like most first-time church visitors, we settled in a straight-backed pew about halfway toward the front. I leaned forward to inventory the pew racks, which were packed with the usual suspects — offering envelopes, visitor registration cards and hymnals.

They were even equipped with the rubber O-rings that Baptist churches have used for decades to soften the clanking sound that empty communion cups can make when returned to uncushioned pews. I was tempted to extract the O-ring and send it bouncing down the pew as I had in my teen years, but the nice usher likely had his eye on me.

Two minutes before the service began, folks were still making small talk about the NBA playoffs or the upcoming church picnic. At 11 a.m., though, the glistening organ pipes shushed the congregants, calling the wandering ones back into the pews they'd likely occupied for years.

A director in a multicolored shirt stood to lead the congregants in singing "Since Jesus Came Into My Heart." Two more hymns followed, each one sandwiched between announcements or prayers. After the third verse of the third hymn, the ushers started passing the offering plates.

The pastor was on vacation, so a retired minister delivered a three-point sermon in the kindhearted tradition of Southern preaching. No brimstone, just thoughtful points. Twenty minutes later, he began inviting potential converts to leave their pews, walk down the aisle and declare before the congregation their intent to be born again.

Now, if you're wondering why I'd interrupt a visit with grandchildren to find my way into a worship service that lacks today's evangelical, chorus-singing drumbeat, I believe it was to recapture a moment.

It was the moment nearly 50 years ago that I released my grip on the pew and walked toward my "Pastor Dad," as he stood before his much-smaller Baptist pulpit outside Monterey, California. In a very public declaration of faith, I wrapped my arms around his waist and told Dad that I wanted to follow Jesus.

My decision caused my face to hurt with the hurt you get from stifling the tears you know will embarrass you. Yet there was nothing overly dramatic in that moment. No "falling down in the spirit," nothing mysterious, new age, mystical or magical. It was a simple, quiet knowing that God was in my heart.

And thankfully, my visit to Walterboro reminded me not only that God has remained in my heart, but also that when it comes to God, you can always go home again.

When recommending a place of worship, I try to consider the needs of the person asking. The request sometimes comes from a new resident, but it often arises from someone I perceive as a "hopper."

Hoppers are discriminate shoppers looking for a perfect worship place. They want a youth group for Johnny, a children's program for Sissy and a nursery with closed-circuit television monitors and daddy-pagers.

They are most happy when they can find a short sermon and a big-band experience. Throw in Big Gulp communion cups and first-class pew legroom and they are ready for the membership class.

Truth be told, I've shopped with similar expectations. I've taken a seat on the back pew with the frustration of a benched quarterback wondering things like, "Where did this guy get his degree?" Or, "Does she really think she can pull off a 45-minute sermon? Or, "Is he going to quit preaching before the nodding parishioner cracks his skull on the pew?"

Maybe I should give hoppers some credit. At least they make the effort to find a place to belong. Some folks don't see the point in searching for a worship place at all. They believe they can have a spiritual life without a spiritual community. They often tell me they see too many hypocrites at church.

To that common complaint I'm always tempted to say, "Don't worry, I'm sure they can make room for another hypocrite." Hold your e-mails. I just think it; I don't say it.

Instead, I encourage folks to see the unique quality in faith communities. Unique in that they remain the only gathering place in the world where people assemble for the sole purpose of publicly acknowledging their imperfections.

I like to explain it this way: If you visit a service club such as the Lions or Kiwanis, you'll hear their members brag about being part of the best club in the world. Well they should. These are fine organizations.

Within the community of faith, however, you'll find just the opposite. You'll often hear people who admit they're fatally flawed — all sinners in need of a higher power other than themselves.

If I ever pastor a church again, I have an idea of how a perfect worship experience would begin. I'd start it much the same way Alcoholics Anonymous begins their meeting. I'd instruct the congregants to form a single-file line to the lectern.

Once in front of the microphone, each would take a turn saying something like, "Hi, I'm Norris and I'm a sinner, big time." I suggest this little liturgy because I've discovered that when you begin worship from the place of your own imperfections, you will be blessed with the deepest insights.

That's a truth I've known ever since I wrote my first F-word with that broken sheetrock to say, "Dennis is a big *fink*."

I was such a creative writer, even then.

Putting Gratitude in our Faith

As a hospital chaplain, I work in a secular world. I see and hear a lot of amazing miracles, but I also hear the vulgar on a regular basis. I once was about to exit a visit with a hospital patient with a nasty infection when the nurse noticed I hadn't followed the hand washing protocol.

"No, no, no, chaplain, you'd better wash those hands before you go in there."

"Yes, ma'am" I said.

"That's right" she said, "You don't want to be on my s*** list."

While I don't identify with the vulgarity, I do identify with the sentiment. I had to confess that I had recently composed such a list of people who'd displeased me.

I know. Tisk, tisk. I'm a chaplain, and I'm not supposed to carry a list like that. Truthfully, though, I was angry with several people involved in a predicament. My natural inclination was to compose an S-list. Then, I remembered what a friend in recovery had told me: Anyone can make an S-list, but few people know how to make a Gratitude list.

I remembered he had challenged me to spend a half hour in prayer composing a list of all I was grateful for — a G-List, so I did. At first I sounded like Tiny Tim, "Thank you for mommy and daddy, and sister and dog — blah, blah." It felt phony and insincere, but the more I worked on the list, the more the list started working on me.

My father taught me a lot about gratitude. He was a pastor who showed a great deal of faith through his practice of gratitude. He was a farmer's son and child of the depression era. He worked hard and instead of enumerating the things he didn't have, he started the day assessing what he did have.

However, there was one thing he was missing that he always seemed grateful not to have – the upper half of his middle finger.

He always seemed to be grateful that it was missing. Strange viewpoint, right? Yes, it was. That strange viewpoint came out of a factory accident he had while working part time to pay for theological school.

That evening, he came home to my mother with his left hand wrapped tightly in a bloodied bandage. He had been processing books into a binding machine when he got too close and severed half of his middle finger. There was no reattaching a finger in the rural town hosting the plant, and he would have to adapt to the loss.

After he died, I reflected on the many ways in which he learned to adapt, and even thrive, with his minor physical impairment.

Professionally, he knew his oddly shaped hand might distract a church parishioner, so his gestures minimized the obvious gap.

Socially, if someone expressed sympathy and asked about his missing finger half, he never skipped a beat joking that my mother bit it off.

Physically, he thrived, because the finger worked like a second thumb, which gave him a vice-like grip for his part-time work as an electrician.

And spiritually, he used it best to love his children.

The love usually began on Saturday night after watching WWF wrestling on our black-and-white TV. My siblings and I would leap onto my father's back and entangle him with 12 skinny arms and legs. I usually began the ambush by hopping on his chest, while my brother twisted his arms and my sister yanked on his prematurely balding head.

Pretending to be overwhelmed with us, he'd suddenly announce the arrival of his secret weapon. That's what he called his dwarfed middle finger when deploying it as the most pernicious tickling device known to kid-kind.

"No! Not fair!" we'd scream as he zeroed in on our most vulnerable ticklish spots with his stealthy, stubby, silly weapon. When he grew tired of the tickling, he'd morph the "weapon" into a thumping device upon our chest, "torturing" us with it until we rolled off his side.

Was it really a secret weapon? Or was it a just a half of a finger? Or was it a communication device that delivered a spiritual connection of love for his children?

I guess the answer to that question is at the fingertip of the user, but on my father's hand, it was a weapon of endearing love that he used to amuse, engage and disarm people.

In the grown-up world that I must now live, people routinely use that finger to cast a vulgar curse toward the existence of another. They use it as the gavel of random judgment. They use it to dehumanize another. They use it to offend.

There's an interesting verse in the Christian Scripture commanding us to cut off any body part that offends. "If your right hand offends you," Jesus says, "cut it off."

While interpretations vary, no scholar would suggest literal amputation. But, oddly enough, when I read that Scripture, I sometimes think of my father's finger.

When a youthful accident removed half of his cursing finger, he created something that was a source of humor and strength, and more important, he transformed it into a pipeline that delivered his love into the souls of his giggling children.

At the end of his life of 65 short years, his middle finger had been transformed into something less a curse and much more of a blessing he was grateful for. It's a view of the finger the world could use more of and I still sorely miss.

As I continued to build my gratitude list, I was reminded of a question routinely asked by the minister of music in a church I pastored. He'd stand behind the big Baptist pulpit and ask this question of his sleepy and aging congregation:

"Would you rather be in the best prison in America or here in church today?"

He used the question to roust our aging congregation and inspire them to sing louder. He often used it at the Thanksgiving service because he felt like it gave congregants a bit of gratitude perspective. The reasoning is a bit haggard as it's the same kind of sermonic reasoning ministers use every year that urge us to remember those less fortunate.

I ask you, can't we just hold the guilt this year and sit back and relax with our holiday pie?

Newspaper columnists like myself, and most especially ministers, of whom I am both, try to make you see that your life is not as bad as it could be. This approach comes off sounding a lot like a parent trying to get their kid to eat turnips. "At least we have turnips and broccoli on our table," goes the paternal reasoning, "I'll bet the kids in Godawfulstan wish they had turnips." That line of reasoning never did much for me.

The problem with that perspective is that gratitude and thankfulness has never been about comparing your good fortune to the misfortunes of others. Thanksgiving will never be about trying to equalize the imbalance of those fortunes.

Thanksgiving isn't just about being grateful you don't have a loved one deployed to a war-torn country. It's also about being thankful we have brave service members who are willing to serve when their country calls.

Thanksgiving isn't just about being grateful you aren't poor. It is also about being grateful you have resources to give to the poor.

It is not only about being grateful you aren't hungry. It is also about sharing your gratitude with the hungry.

Being truly thankful is not about comparing what you have with what others do not have. It is not about being glad your home is not a shanty cardboard shack under the freeway. It's about the help we give the homeless as we humbly realize that most of us are one paycheck away from building our own shack.

Gratitude is not about giving thanks for what you have, where you work, where you live or even who you are. Thanksgiving is not about you at all.

Thanksgiving is about keeping perspective between recognizing the blessings we've received and utilizing our capacity to return those blessings to others.

At the end of the calorie-laden day, perspective will be a constant reminder that we are not alone on this planet. It is the perspective of gratitude that teaches us we've all journeyed from the same place and, as Scripture suggests, "to dust we will return."

That is the perspective from which humility comes, and humility will always be about gratitude.

I often feel ungrateful as expressed in the two prayers I feel some shame for praying. The first prayer starts off with, "God, please make me like this man." I pray this prayer when I hear from friends such as Cecil Murphy, who tells me his New York Times best-selling book, "90 Minutes in Heaven," just surpassed 3 million in sales.

It's a prayer I pray in the midst of people such as Andy Petruska. Andy's a retired U.S. Navy captain who still is navigating the seven seas with his wife, Laura, as merchant marines. I often stay in their Florida home and swap his sea stories for my less-than-exciting chaplain stories well into the night.

Oh, I know what you're thinking. Those are self-defeating prayers, Norris. Don't say things like that. Well, like you, I pray these prayers because I'm human.

Regretfully, the most human prayer I pray is the "At Least Prayer."

It starts like this: "Thank you, God, that at least I'm not as bad as so-and-so!"

No, it's not a prayer I vocalize. It's a prayer that slips from the surly bonds of my brain and erupts when I'm asked for change by the fourth homeless person of the day. "Thank you, God, that at least I work for a living."

Or it comes out when I browse a lousy book and I say, "At least I can write."

Or it erupts at the gas station when some fellow pulls in driving a Hummer with his stereo blasting. The self-serving jerk is yelling into his tiny wireless earpiece about some business deal gone bad, all the while pretending he doesn't notice the single mom who's been waiting 10 minutes for the spot he took.

The prayer slips into my conscious stream of thought through an un-spoken barrel roll of my eyes. "Thank you, God, I'm not like him!"

Maybe you're praying it now. "Thank God I'm not like this hypocriti-cal chaplain!"

Maybe I should be a better example of what Chuang Tzu, a Chinese philosopher who lived during the fourth century B.C, described. "The Perfect Man has no self; the Holy Man has no merit; the Sage has no fame." (Chuang Tzu, 26).

But you'd have to admit we tend to think this way. For instance, did you say it to the cop who ticketed you last month? "At least I don't weave through traffic!"

Have you said it to your children when they've complained about your overbearing attitude? "At least I let you go the movies."

The thinking is similar to a man Jesus described in Luke 18. He stood praying in the front of the temple when he noticed over his shoulder a Roman collaborator, the most hideous of all beings.

"Thank you God that I am not like thissss man," he hissed.

His At Least Prayer was so loud, he failed to hear the prayer of the one he condemned.

The message translation says the man "slumped in the shadows, his face in his hands, not daring to look up, saying, 'God, give mercy. Forgive me, a sinner.' "

"Jesus commented, 'This tax man, not the other, went home, made right with God.' "

Then Jesus said something that will forever squelch the At Least Prayer.

"If you walk around with your nose in the air, you're going to end up flat on your face, but if you're content to be simply yourself, you will be-come more than yourself."

I work to be grateful for the time I have. This is the lesson of the miniature grandfather's clock in my living room. It has this simple way of harassing me about the writing deadlines that threaten my daily bliss.

Everything is going well until each additional bell reminds me that an hour has slipped by without accomplishment. Hemingway may be right, and the bell may toll for me, but what is the intent of its persistence?

Is it a bell that seduces me into my future? Or is the bell dragging me into, and nagging me about, my past failures?

Or perhaps the bell serves as a foghorn beseeching me to remain on the course set by the moment.

If so, I hear the bell announcing: "Be grateful for this is the moment you are given. This is your time. There'll be no others."

In fact, not to be gloomy, but the chimes ask a very scriptural question: "For what is your life? It is even as a vapor."

The chimes remind me that life will end shortly and will take with it any chances I have of making this moment into something meaningful.

So to risk a cliché, I use the bell to ask myself, "What would I do if I knew this bell was the prelude to my funeral dirge?"

Asked properly, even the common tasks are blessed with new significance.

What might I eat? What might I read? Would I finally let Toby, my pesky pound puppy, soak my face with his salivating tongue?

If I knew this bell signaled my final round in my fight for life, would I become an ambassador for peace? Would I stage a sit-in to protest the war and end my midnight chaplain visits that carry the "regrets of the secretary of the Army"?

If it were my last bell, whom would I love? Whose forgiveness would I seek? To whom would I grant grace? Would I use the moments to make peace with a child who is finding no peace about her future?

Would I tell my aging mother I love her more than once? Or would I make certain that my brother, who displays many of the symptoms of Asperger's syndrome, knows that God has always loved him just the way he is and so do I?

As we read these words today, we are among the fortunate who have heard the next bell. Welcome to our future. We are here.

Now the question is, what has God blessed you with? What are you thankful for? And will you share these blessings with gratitude?

I believe this is what my clock is asking. It's not harassing me for busting a deadline, and it's not enticing me into a future. It's saying that we've arrived in the now. This moment is all we are promised. It's time to live it.

I am always grateful for food. In fact I've often joked that potlucks are among the main reasons I became a minister. Apparently I'm not alone in my culinary reverence for feasting because when I gather with fellow clergy, we do what most of us do all too well — eat.

Like many Thanksgiving potlucks, ours began when the Methodist minister who chairs our gatherings invited us to share something for which we're thankful.

A Pentecostal colleague began by broadcasting the dramatic news of his church's numerical growth. A young Congregational pastor followed him, telling of her husband's new job. Another pastor stood to share a story of forgiveness that his congregation had extended to an erring staff member.

As most people looked around wondering who'd be next, I stared into my empty plate. I wanted to share how grateful I was that someone brought deviled eggs, but thought better of it.

Then, just as our convener was signaling the beginning of our meal with a raised fork, a priest from Sierra Leone cleared his throat.

"I am thankful that Ebola has come to America," he said.

There was a sudden stillness in the room, quickly broken by the retired priest seated next to me.

"Father!" exclaimed the retiree, "How can you be thankful for such a horrible thing?"

The priest, not a man to be shamed, stood and took a clearing breath before answering, "Ebola has been infecting our people for at least 10 years, yet America has only seen Ebola as a minor thing."

As he sat back down, he added, "I'm grateful that America now seems motivated to find a cure."

Most of us responded with stunned silence, staring at the 40-something priest as though he were a terrorist looking to propagate the infection.

But, in the few moments that followed the awkward silence, I heard the understanding tones of "hmm" and "ohhh" spreading through our gathering.

We got it. With one short stab, the priest had proclaimed the unspeakable and rightfully chastened us for our country's lack of action.

His words brought to mind a saying I often hear in our surgical department: "Minor surgery is what happens to you. Major surgery is what happens to me." While we are truly the most generous nation in the world, it seems as though it wasn't until the disease reached our shores that we saw it as anything more than a minor problem.

The priest reminded us that what happens to a piece of our world is happening to the whole. When it comes to Ebola, there are no first, second and third worlds.

There's only one world and there's no escape from it. NASA isn't going to transport us to a massive space station or repopulate us to another planet. The president isn't writing an executive order to build a quarantine wall around our coasts. If we don't survive together, we will die together.

Ebola is the strangest thing I've ever heard someone express thanks for, but by the end of our thankful meal, the priest's remark had reminded us of the wisdom from Luke 12:48, "To whom much is given, much shall be required."

During the holidays, as you say a prayer of thanks, stop for a minute and ask yourself a question. If we are truly thankful for all God has provided in our lives, aren't we also responsible to share those provisions with others?

Building a Thriving Faith with Prayer

When I meet people with a thriving faith, they are not only grateful people, but they are also prayerful people. That's why I see prayer as the second aspect of faith. Prayer means many different things to many different cultures. Prayer is sometimes confused with meditation. They aren't the same, but they might well be two sides of the same coin. Prayer is talking to God. Meditation is listening to God. As in any good conversation, we must listen and talk.

However, most people are nervous about beginning that conversation. After all, we are talking to GOD. So, what do we say? How do we start?

Mr. Penny was asking the same questions when he asked his nurse to find the chaplain. I call him "mister" because that's how he formally introduced himself at the Houston Northwest Medical Center in 1992.

Perhaps he meant the "mister" title to formalize the relationship between young and old, but my guess was that he meant to distance himself from his stereotypical idea of the "preacher."

Penny had inoperable brain cancer, but he didn't want to talk about that. The balding, bony man steered most of our conversations to things like his opinion of the Houston Oilers and my lunchtime basketball games with local clergy.

Over the next several months, Penny was admitted a half dozen more times, but on his last hospitalization his nurse summoned me from lunch. "Mr. Penny" had a favor he wanted to ask.

Thinking his request sounded like the call to a deathbed confession, I made a quick exit from the cafeteria and hurried to ICU. I walked into the room to find Mrs. Penny stroking her husband's fevered head. "Oh good," she said. "I'm glad you're here, but I thought Tuesday was your basketball day." "Knee problems," I said, patting my left knee.

She exhaled in relief.

"He wants to ask you something," she said. I looked at the figure on the bed, twisted and ghostly. His raspy breathing suggested he wouldn't have much strength for this conversation, so I leaned over the bed and called to him as if announcing my presence through a dense fog.

"Mr. Penny, it's Chaplain Norris," I said. "Is there something you want to ask me?" He nodded.

"Teach me," he said, his voice trailing off. He took a fuller breath and added, "Teach me to pray." I searched his wife's face for context. She chewed at her thumbnail as she explained that her husband was embarrassed to ask for God's help at such a late hour.

"He's afraid he's being hypocritical," she added.

I often hear this reasoning from patients, and it always reminds me of the two revolutionaries who died on the crosses beside Jesus. The first man spent his last hours mocking Jesus and goading him to use his magical powers to save everyone.

The other guy was quite the opposite. He felt shame for his past life, so he asked Jesus, "Remember me when you enter your kingdom." Instead of disqualifying the man for being hypocritically late, Jesus assured him that he would see his new spiritual home that very day.

"Mr. Penny," I said. "I think you'll find that God cares very little about your past. He mostly cares what you'll do with the next minute of your life." Penny nodded.

"Prayer is just talking to God. It's not theologically complicated," I added. "Just talk from your heart." Penny closed his eyes and began moving his lips.

I couldn't hear what he was saying, but when he opened his eyes his expression told me that he'd heard God's voice. I know this because the "mister" who had originally sought to distance himself from spiritual matters managed to say one last thing to me.

"Thank you, pastor. Thank you."

Not all my patients have been so appreciative. Five years ago, I was working as a hospital chaplain at Sutter Medical Center in Sacramento when a nurse suggested I visit one of her patients.

The busy nurse offered little reason for her referral, only that our patient might need "some counseling or something." Before entering the room, I found more explanation in the patient's chart, which said he was consuming multiple six-packs each day.

"Yup or 'something,' " I muttered, repeating the nurse's euphemism.

Inside the room, I met a man who was writhing in the pain of detoxification. From what little I know about the process, it makes waterboarding look tame.

Fixing me with a crazed look, he ordered me to "Get some &%@'n drugs, doc!" He was, no doubt, assuming that a male wearing a necktie was his doctor.

I took a deep breath and assured him I was his chaplain, not his doctor

Arming himself again with a limited vocabulary, he fired another volley aimed at convincing me he didn't care whether I was the pope; he wanted his drugs.

I nodded and left the room to relay his message to the nurse.

"Did you tell him that he shouldn't talk to a chaplain that way?" she asked.

My forthcoming answer seemed to shock her nearly as much as the patient's language.

"No. I think his language represents a kind of prayer."

"Prayer?" she asked, with a look that said she was questioning my sobriety.

I took her stance as invitation to say more. In the next few minutes, I shared my belief that God hears our expressions of agony, loss or pain as a prayer.

These prayers can be expressed in a wordless whimper, and God hears them. They can be said with bloodcurdling screams, and God hears them. They are even vented with words that will offend the offhanded listener. The point is that no matter how these words are said, God hears them and knows how to interpret them.

Our problem often comes when, like the nurse, we close our hearts and our ears to the kind of language expressed in that level of pain. We do this because we think pain ought not become offensive. "Pain should be neat and controlled," we reason.

That's not the way the Psalmist saw it when he wrote, "I cry aloud to the Lord; I lift up my voice to the Lord for mercy. I pour out my complaint before him; before him I tell my trouble." (Psalm 142:1-2)

And it certainly wasn't the way Job saw it when he lost his entire family. "Therefore I will not keep silent; I will speak out in the anguish of my spirit, I will complain in the bitterness of my soul." (Job 7:11)

I'm not saying we should encourage this language in everyday use. I'm saying that if God doesn't turn his ears away from even the most excruciating levels of human pain, then how can we?

At the end of the day, I like the metaphor Susan Lenzkes uses in her book, "When Life Takes What Matters." She says expressing our anger is like beating upon the chest of God, but "… We beat on His chest from within the circle of His arms."

I came back to see the man a few hours later and found him apologetic for his language, but thankful his nurse had heard his "prayer."

"If talking to God is just talking," you ask. "Then whom do we pray for first?"

I recently found that answer during one of my cross-country speaking jaunts. It came to me as listened to the flight attendant's safety speech: "If you are traveling with children, or are seated next to someone who needs assistance, place the mask on yourself first, then offer assistance."

As a chaplain it seems counterintuitive to put myself before all others. But I know that it's strategic advice to save myself first so I am able to help save others.

As ironic at that advice seems, it's solid counsel – especially when it comes to prayer. In fact, it's guidance I give every week during the spirituality group I conduct inside a locked psychiatric facility.

The group is composed of fewer than a dozen inpatients from various religious and nonreligious backgrounds. Because of those varied backgrounds, the group isn't the Bible study you might expect from a pastor.

Nevertheless, we delve into some spiritual resources from a page of powerful faith quotes from the likes of Billy Graham, Helen Keller, Martin Luther King and others.

I close the group by asking participants, "What are you praying for yourself?" (I allow the nonreligious to supply their own verb: "hoping, seeking, desiring, etc.)

"This can't be a prayer for Aunt Mary or a new car," I say. "In your heart of hearts, tell me what you personally seek from God?"

Invariably, most respond with a single word like, "sobriety, peace, forgiveness, direction and contentment."

I know it sounds outlandish for a chaplain to suggest that you pray for yourself before praying for others, but there's rhyme to my reason.

And it's this. In the book, "God for the 21st Century," Dale Mathews contributed a chapter called Faith and Medicine in which he cites university studies investigating the efficacy of two kinds of prayer: Intercessory Prayer (praying for others) and Petitionary Prayer (praying for yourself.)

Mathews admits that praying for others is hard to measure. He cites research done by Dr. Harold Koenig, an associate professor of medicine at Duke University and the country's leading authority on faith-and-medicine studies.

Koenig found that "…in studies of intercessory prayer where one person prays for the health of another, there is scant if any effect." Now please don't think I'm arguing that prayer doesn't work; it just doesn't lend itself to laboratory studies.

However, Koenig found that "…in the studies of petitionary prayer where a person prays for his or her own health or peace of mind there were tangible and quantifiable results."

Amazingly, he says, "When you pray for your own health–especially your own mental health, … science suggests you may be on solid ground."

The study has caused me to urge patients to pray for themselves before praying for that errant grandson. Before praying for a new job, perhaps pray for yourself. Before praying that your spouse will stop drinking, pray for yourself.

Does that seem selfish? I don't think so. I see a cogent parallel between the flight attendant asking you to tend to yourself and me asking you to pray for yourself.

Maybe the time we spend praying to become the creation God intends us to be is God's way of helping everyone around us – the helpless, the hapless, the homeless, the sick and wounded journeying beside us in our flight through this world.

So this week I encourage you to voice prayers for yourself. And while you do, my prayer will be that whatever miracle you seek from God's hand will begin with the changes he makes in you.

At this time, you may return your seats to the upright position and remember that your baggage may have shifted during the reading of this book.

If praying for oneself seems awkward, then you should try praying for someone you haven't met. Consider my prayer for a patient I've never met and will probably never meet. He's more than likely dead.

I only know about him at all because Ken, the affable nurse who schedules our hospital surgeries, left me a voicemail saying that a patient was requesting prayer prior to his scheduled surgery the following week.

So, early on the following Monday, I went to the presurgery holding area to pray with the patient. The only problem was that he wasn't there and the surgical staff didn't seem to have any idea who I was talking about.

The confusion sent me back to Ken.

"Oh, sorry," he said, "I meant to leave you a follow-up message letting you know that the doctors canceled the surgery. Our patient has pancreatitis, infection of the pancreas."

"Can't that be fixed?" I asked.

"Yup, but the pancreatitis was only the symptom of the real problem. The guy has pancreatic cancer. He's done. The docs told him to stay home and just be comfortable with his family."

"So there's no hope?" I asked.

"Nope. It's so sad because the guy's only 30. I've only seen one guy recover from that, and it was a genuine miracle."

Then Ken added, "I guess you can always pray for a miracle."

Taking Ken's suggestion, I found a quiet place where I made an honest effort to honor the patient's request for prayer on that particular day.

I must confess that the prayer felt awkward. The patient was a total stranger to me. It reminded me of the times I'd been in church when someone asked for prayer for an obscure or unfamiliar situation, like someone's Aunt Sally in Timbuktu. Those prayer requests were easy to slough off because they didn't directly affect me.

My prayerful effort called to mind the words of a song written by Ty Lacy and Steve Siler called "Not Too Far From Here."

> "Somebody's down to their last dime
> Somebody's running out of time
> Not too far from here
> Somebody's got nowhere else to go
> Somebody needs a little hope
> Not too far from here
>
> "And I may not know their name
> But I'm praying just the same
> That you'll use me, Lord
> To wipe away the tears
> 'Cause somebody's crying
> Not too far from here"

Those lyrics express the truth that we will not always have a front row seat to God's plans or be able to see the closing act of what God has in mind. That shouldn't keep us from praying for all those in need of prayer.

So, though I knew nothing about the patient beyond what I'd learned from Ken, I did what he requested. I prayed. I prayed that he would be wrapped in the loving care of his family. I prayed that he'd be able to finish his business on earth. And I prayed for a miracle that wasn't definable in human terms.

So, the next time you're feeling helpless or awkward at being asked to pray for someone you don't know or for a situation that is far removed from you, I hope you'll find inspiration in the song's last verse to do so:

> "Now I'm letting down my guard
> And I'm opening my heart
> Help me speak your love
> To every needful ear
> Someone is waiting
> Not too far from here"

Once we pray for ourselves, and then pray for those we don't know, we turn our prayers to people we do know.

However, the problem is, how do we know what to pray for them.

Just ask them.

"Isn't that forward or kind of presumptive?" you ask.

Not at all. Consider how many times a day you ask the question, "How are you?"

Each time you ask, someone will likely respond, "fine."

Really? Are we always fine?

We go to church, support groups or mother's house for Thanksgiving and proclaim that we are fine. Then we turn to the next person to repeat the question.

What a coincidence. Everyone is fine.

Recently, I've begun substituting that question with a new one.

This past week, I challenged audiences in Florida, Colorado and Ohio to make the same substitution and ask, "What have you been praying for?"

If the word prayer is too religious, the alternate approach is to ask people what they are hoping for (or visualizing.)

I first started asking the question earlier this year with the encourage-ment of a hospital colleague named chaplain Gerald Jones. When visiting patients, he gives them a chance to breach the mundane and to share their heart's desire.

There are a few who'll respond with the stereotypical answer of a beauty contestant and proclaim they are praying for world peace.

But most will answer it with the kind of honesty I heard earlier this year from a woman facing her pending death.

She was leaving high school-age children and was praying everyone would find some kind of meaning in her death.

Afterwards, I went to my computer and paraphrased our visit into a prayer. After I wrote it, I offered this prayer as a gift.

God,

There may be those who think I should be mad at you; I need you to know it's nothing like that. I know things like this happen in a world you created, and there is no purpose in being mad at you.

In fact — and this is the crazy thing — I actually think you've given me a gift. It's the gift of seeing. I now see what was always there. Now I see the wonderful network of friends and family you have put here to help me. I feel your hands through their caring hands. I know your love through their protective love. Thank you for this gift.

There's a road ahead of me that I cannot see, and that's OK. It's OK because you can see it, and you've got it taken care of. It's OK because my life has always belonged to you. You created me and you sustain me. You take care of me the way I love my children.

Speaking of children, that's my only worry. I know they cope with things differently because you blessed them with their own individual personalities.

But, I also need to know that you take care of them. Hold them in your hands and help them to cope. Help them see the blessing of family that you have given us. Help them see that this blessing is the only thing that will sustain us through this difficult time.

Thank you for your love for me. May I be a light that shines with your love.

Amen.

I left our visit with a new perspective.

So, today I challenge you to ask one person what they are praying for. I think, you'll find what I found. In a time that finds us so divided, this simple question has a powerful potential to bring us together.

"Can I pray for you?" asked a pushy pastor who pressed his way into my chaplain's office one day. He seemed determined to introduce himself and bless me with his famous presence, so I let him talk.

I knew things would get interesting when he introduced himself as the spirit-filled "Brother So-and-So." If you are unfamiliar with the adjective "Spirit-filled," it means to embody the spirit of Christ. Or, loosely translated, it's the charismatic next step after "born-again."

Let me pause a moment to say, I have lots of wonderful charismatic friends. And most of them will tell you that if you are indeed filled with the Spirit, there is no need to self-identify as such. If true, it will be obvious.

Suffice it to say, I was quickly wishing that Mr. Brother Pastor had kept walking the hall. But instead, the tall, broad and aging pastor sat down and proceeded to recite his resume.

He talked about the prison ministry he ran and he fed me the details of his meals to the homeless. He buzzed about the radio preaching he did in Fresno and the television ministry he ran in Bakersfield.

In between each story, he paused to wait for my "amen," but alas, I offered only a polite nod. He talked so long and so fast, I was having trouble hearing the Spirit.

He then shifted the conversation into the many years he served as a pastor and the hospital visitations he did. He confessed that he pitied me because "we both know that government chaplains can't talk about God as freely as a pastor."

And somewhere in the midst of his pontification, he told me that he was praying that God would make him "teachable." If he noticed the smirk that word "teachable" brought to my face, he didn't say.

Instead, he abruptly assumed a crouching position and announced that he was going to pray for me. That's when I decided that I'd answer his prayer and offer him a teachable moment.

"Wait just a minute," I said. "How do you know what to pray for?"

"Huh?" he asked.

I asked this because people sometimes offer their prayers, not as a gift, but as a way to establish their power over the pray-ee. My guess was that Pastor Pray4U was going to thank God that I was blessed by his visit today.

I continued. "Well, you mentioned a few minutes ago that you were praying God would make you teachable, so let me share something with you."

He gave me a glassy stare, as clueless as a calf frozen before a new gate.

"When I visit a patient, I always ask them how I can pray for them. I ask them what they want me to pray for. Wouldn't you like to know what you can pray for me?"

With that, God answered his prayer to become teachable and he leaned back in his chair, and spread his hands open on his lap.

"You're right," he said. "What should I pray?"

I asked that he pray for our incoming chaplain supervisor and our new chapel. He agreed with a humble nod. Then I asked him to pray that God would comfort the families of the two hospital employees who'd unexpectedly died the previous week.

He shook his head, still unsure what to say.

He did pray, just not the prayer I'd expected. His prayer was a humble and contrite one asking God for the things we agreed upon. After he'd said the "amen," he raised his head and our eyes met. This time I read a "spirit filled" look that indeed told me he just might be teachable.

If you really don't know what to pray, you'd do well to review the principles of prayer found in the Lord's Prayer, or as biblical scholars call it, "The Model Prayer."

While I use the prayer year round, it particularly says a lot to me during the holiday shopping frenzy that follows Thanksgiving. By the first of December, Thanksgiving is just a speed bump in our memory as we race toward the Black Friday sales.

If this holiday track meet leaves you frazzled, I want to offer you a choice of two very different running lanes. First, you can align yourself with denial and tell yourself that you're overspending so that you'll have more to be thankful for next year.

Choice number 2 is to pause before you get trapped in the StuffMart or CostlyCo aisles and recite what I like to call the Black Friday prayer. While you'll likely recognize the prayer as "The Lord's Prayer," let's reframe it to see how it might be said to rescue us from our manic materialism.

The opening salutation, "Our Father," is best read in the tone of a small child who is asking a loving parent for help. The words assert that God alone is the giver of all good things, not credit cards.

"Who art in heaven." These words may sound like a description of a detached deity, but in truth, God contains the world. That means that our money can't buy our world, so why do we try?

"Hallowed be thy name." There seems little that is hallowed today, but when we find that hallowedness in God, it should reflect something outside of our own name and holiday wish lists.

"Thy Kingdom come" doesn't mean that we're sitting around waiting for God to come to us. It means that we must invite the presence of God into our own lives. It means that God's presence always outshines the pretense of presents.

"Thy will be done, on Earth as it is in Heaven."

This part means that seeking God's will in my life is not seeking an earthly plan. Simply put, I've never seen a U-Haul trailer hooked to a hearse, so I don't think God wants me to accumulate much more earthly goods than are useful for heavenly purposes. Reciting this part of the prayer makes it nearly impossible to exceed your credit card limit.

"Give us this day our daily bread." The recovering alcoholic knows this as the key to living "one day at a time," but the recovering shopper should see this as a way to express gratitude for the gifts we find in today, not the presents we'll return tomorrow.

"Forgive us our trespasses as we forgive those who trespass against us." This plea for forgiveness reminds me that God forgives me my selfish ways and that my overspending transgressions of the past, don't have to be repeated today.

"Lead us not into temptation, but deliver us from evil." This phrase reminds me that I am powerless before my shopping addictions, and I can only overcome them with God's help.

While Protestants add the closing line, "For thine is the Kingdom, the power, the glory, forever," both Catholic and Protestants end with 'Amen,' which means, "Let all of this be so!"

Prayer seems like a superstitious practice to some, so I must say that I'm not a superstitious person. However, I've occasionally been passed off as the spiritual equivalent to a rabbit's foot.

One of those occasions happened at Patrick Air Force Base while I served as the launch crew chaplain at nearby Cape Canaveral (1999-2002). In that role, I gave the official prayers for most launches, which included shuttles and satellites.

In military tradition, my prayers were more ceremonial than a legitimate attempt to court God's favor. They were generic in nature, seeking good weather, safety and success.

It's normal for technical difficulties to delay launches, but in the late months of 1999, we had favorable results in launching on our first attempt. Crews began to tie these successes with the arrival of their new chaplain. Their thinking became so ridiculous that one superstitious commander actually checked with my boss to confirm that I'd be the chaplain delivering "their prayer."

These were the same folks who, in good fun, wore something for good luck on every launch day. They brought everything from lucky socks to coins or even a piece of a failed rocket. Now I'd suddenly become their "lucky charm chaplain."

But my luck wasn't going to hold.

One evening, after I'd been there for about six months, I composed a fervent prayer for a 2 a.m. launch. At the last minute, the mission was scrubbed because of weather, but rescheduled for the same time on the next morning.

"God speed," I said, with a dismissive assumption that my job was done.

They looked at me as if I'd hung them with their lucky necktie. "You're coming back tomorrow night, aren't you Chaplain?"

"Uh, sure."

The next morning, I reported for duty, bleary-eyed, hoping to pass off the same crumpled prayer from the previous evening.

Same result. No launch.

As I offered condolences to the disappointed crew, Brigadier General Donald Pettit, the Wing Commander, barked at me. "Chaplain, your prayer didn't work! You need to write a new prayer."

It's possible that what I said next might explain why I had to finish my military career in the reserves.

"You're kidding, sir."

He assured me in general-like terms that he wasn't kidding.

I still thought he was ribbing me, but I was too new to our spacey business to be sure. So, a few days later, I brought a new prayer. Unfortunately for all concerned, I was forced to repeat the rewrites for the next three weeks.

When our rocket finally soared on our sixth attempt, I reached across the consoles to exchange handshakes with the ground crew. One engineer in his lucky sweater, slapped my back and said, "You finally did it, Chaplain."

"Did what?" I wondered, as I drove home on that early morning.

I wasn't the lucky horseshoe in this arrangement. I simply offered a prayer — not as a magical incantation, but as a reminder that God comes where he is invited.

The next morning, I was walking across the base courtyard, when Gen. Pettit motioned me over to him.

I offered him a salute weakened by fatigue.

"Your prayer didn't work!" he said.

"But, sir, I saw it launch."

"We launched it, but it never reached the intended orbit," he said.

"That'll be all," he added, before returning my salute with a smirk that told me he really was ribbing me.

The hardest prayer to pray on this planet is probably the prayer Jesus asks his followers to pray for their enemies. It begs the question that when Jesus commanded his followers to "love your enemies and pray for those who persecute you," was he also thinking of those who are trying to kill you?

That was the question we faced at the combat hospital where I served in 2009 in Balad, Iraq. Our rules of engagement were to treat all patients: U.S. service members, civilians and even enemy combatants.

One day in March 2009, those rules were severely tested when our hospital received two critical patients. The first was a U.S. soldier with a bullet lodged in his head. The other patient was an insurgent who was stable, a tourniquet skillfully applied to his leg wound.

The trauma team found that the soldier had sustained what appeared to be a fatal injury. Most stateside hospitals would have dismissed him with comfort measures and prepared the family for a death.

But not this hospital, not this staff.

They went full-court press and sent the soldier into the operating room where our neurosurgeon searched for the bullet. When she found it, she announced what she'd likely known before surgery: the wound was inoperable.

The soldier wouldn't make it, so they called for their chaplain. I donned a mask, gown and gloves and pushed my way through the swinging OR doors.

Immediately, I was overwhelmed by the remnants of an all-out effort. Tubes, IVs, bags of blood, bandages and pharmacological equipment and monitors were strewn about the room. The rusty smell of blood was impossible to dismiss.

The staff paced the room, leaving bloody stains that traced their sacred struggle to save a life. I didn't have to bring God to the OR, he had long preceded me. His footprints were everywhere to prove it.

Then I saw something I will never forget. Blood was pouring from the soldier's head like a faucet. For a moment I held my breath, but the surgeon resuscitated me with a request.

"Chap! Our boy isn't going to make it. Can you say a few words?"

I breathed again and found a prayer to reach a grieving staff. After saying my "amen," someone sarcastically suggested I should also pray for the insurgent in the adjoining operating room.

The insurgent with the bullet in his leg was a sniper, and he'd likely caused this carnage. Now that man was receiving the best medical care possible from the same people who were grieving the loss of their fellow soldier.

You learn a lot when you care for your friends, but you learn a great deal more when you care for your enemies. As I heard one of the doctors say, "This is Geneva Convention 101," in reference to the requirement to treat wounded combatants.

Jesus summed it all up in the Sermon on the Mount: "You're familiar with the old written law, 'Love your friend,' and its unwritten companion, 'Hate your enemy'?

"I'm challenging that," Jesus flatly stated. "I'm telling you to love your enemies. ... If all you do is love the lovable, do you expect a bonus? Anybody can do that. If you simply say hello to those who greet you, do you expect a medal? Any run-of-the-mill sinner does that." (The Message, Matthew 43-44, 47).

This trauma team didn't settle for "run of the mill."

And just so you know, neither did the soldier's battle buddies; they were the ones who had skillfully applied the life-saving tourniquet to the enemy combatant.

(Story abridged from my book, **"Hero's Highway"** *Amazon 2015)*

I hear the prayers of patients who are hurting, sick and discouraged. Their private prayers are often so amazing that I've wished I could share them with my readers, but their privacy prevents me from doing so.

I can, however, share the prayers that are written in the public journal in our chapel. Visitors are encouraged to write their prayers in the spiral notebook so others may pray with them.

As you read these prayers, I encourage you to do two things. First, recall similar situations where God answered your prayers and granted his grace. Second, I ask you to offer your own prayer for the writers.

Some of the prayers are simple one-liners, like the short prayer of a child asking, "Lord, help me to be a football player." But most are deeply moving entreaties searching for healing, acceptance and understanding.

One of the writers was earnestly searching for meaning:

"God, or whoever,

I don't know if there is a Creator/God. I only know that my day to leave this life will come. I just hope that the memories of my mother and father will be with me just like my parents were with me the day I was born. If there is a Creator/God, he/she will know that I tried to live my life with a clean heart."

Some of the petitioners, like this one, were clearly scared:

"Dear Lord,

"I need your guidance now. I don't have my mom anymore, so my dad and I are lost. My son and his wife have a sick baby girl. I need you to help us. Please hold my family tight. I love you, dear Father.

"In the name of the Father and Holy Spirit."

Other prayers showed a struggle that no one wants to face:

"Dear Lord,

"Mom's accident crossed your desk and you approved it. Now we have to turn off the ventilator. It's the hardest decision this family has ever made. My sister is hanging on with vain hope. Please help her see the truth and let mom go.

"Mom is your child, Lord. I know she has a mansion waiting for her. The rest of us have peace about letting her go. Please pass that peace on to my sister. Time is a factor, Lord. Finances are a factor, too.

"The life she's living now isn't life. It isn't fair to mom to have to be like she is. Please help my sister to understand that we are all suffering. Give our family the strength to cross this bridge and give mom a peace that only you can give.

Amen."

One writer, likely a caregiver, compared her pain to that of her patients. She expressed the guilt many of us feel when seeing our problems in the light of the tragedy experienced by others:

"Dear God,

"No one I know is dying or suffering, so I need to stop being a baby about my problems. I should be praying for those who truly need love and support. I'm going through a divorce, and I feel depressed all the time. However, I'm grateful for my health, friends and family.

"Please help me overcome this feeling of anguish, loss, anxiety and jealousy. It's not good for my health, and I'm unable to help my patients who truly need it.

Thanks for listening.

"Amen."

Finally, the last page of the prayer anthology pronounces a benediction for this column:

"To anyone who reads this: I hope God answers all your prayers. The Lord is good! Amen."

Are two prayers better than one? Maybe. Recently I met someone who thought so. It's as if she had a "Buy One Get One" coupon, (BOGO) and she wanted to redeem it for a BOGO for prayer.

She was an octogenarian who was admitted into our Cardiac Intensive Care Unit for routine heart tests.

"Good morning," I said, calling her by name. "I'm Norris."

"Hello, doctor." she said. "I've been waiting to see you."

"Oh, I'm not a doctor," I said, with a warm smile. (My neckties often encourage that assumption. I must admit that it's a mistake I sometimes enjoy, if only for a microsecond.)

"I'm the chaplain," I said. I paused for her to process that information and waited for the assumptions that often follow. This is the moment folks either assume I've come to tell them that they are dying or I've come to convert them.

Fortunately, she assumed neither. With a clear, welcoming tone, she asked me to sit down.

As I sat, I invited her to share her faith journey with me. Over the next half hour, she unfolded her lifetime. She'd been raised as a Lutheran in wartime Europe. Her faith had helped her though the hardship of war, her family's immigration and the struggle to earn a living while trying to learn the English language.

Finally, she arrived at the present day in her story. She told me she was praying that her hospital test results would turn out well.

When I asked if I could pray for her, she nodded. "Please pray with me that the tests will help the doctors solve my problems."

Then I asked, as I commonly do, a point of clarification.

"Would you like me to pray for you right now? Or would you like me to add you on to my prayer list that I pray over at the end of my day?" I introduce this option because it allows the patient some latitude and doesn't put them on the spot.

She leaned forward from her pillow to add a question of her own to the mix. "Do you get paid for this job?"

Her question caught me off guard. It had the random tone of a dementia patient. However, this woman was very intentional about what she was asking.

"Yes, ma'am," I said. "The hospital pays me for my work."

"Well, then," she concluded. "I'll expect both."

I released a hesitant chuckle that showed me to be a little slow on the uptake.

"I'm sorry. Both?" I asked.

"I'm answering your question. If you are paid to do this, I want you to say a prayer for me both now and later," she said.

I pointed a finger toward her in the way one does when admitting that a worthy opponent has unmistakably taken the upper ground.

"You got me," I said. "You definitely got me. Yes, I'll pray for you both now and, most certainly, later." This lady was the BOGO champ. She was definitely getting two prayers for the price of one.

She countered with a wry smile at getting the upper hand. We laughed another moment together, then she offered me her hand to hold as I prayed.

That spunky octogenarian came to our hospital with an exhausted heart, but she proved that the heart of her spunk will likely never be exhausted.

Prayers aren't magic, but I did meet an Air Force sergeant who thought they were. She was like the many others I'd counseled during my 28 years as an Air Force chaplain. Her supervisor sent her to my office in hopes of avoiding a career-threatening visit to mental health. That arrangement usually worked well. However, she seemed bent on sabotaging the arrangement.

As she looked around for the right place to sit, she continuously mumbled the same complaint: "My incantations just aren't working."

I wanted to say, "And neither is your attempt to shock the Protestant chaplain," but instead I invited the sergeant to sit across from me and encouraged her to say more.

Over the next 30 minutes she revealed she was a cutter. If you're not familiar with cutting, it's an attempt to cope with emotional pain by deliberately cutting one's body.

As a practicing Wiccan, she told me of her failure to cast the right spell that would stop her cutting urges. Adding to her frustration was her mother, who was threatening to evict her unless she renounced her religion.

"I still practice," she whispered. "I just keep my crystals and candles hidden."

Lest you assume the woman's plight was because of her religious beliefs, you should know that I heard her story echoed in the words of an Apostolic woman the very next week.

I was making my rounds as a chaplain in a Northern California hospital when I met the woman, in her early 30s, who was suffering from a life-shortening disease. In soft sobs, she told me how the Apostolic faith she'd adopted from her parents was failing her.

"My parents blame me for not getting well. They accuse me of praying with a lack of faith. They say I'm not believing God will heal me."

I was hearing the same motif. The woman used different words than my Wiccan visitor used, but she was expressing the same thought.

Both women were voicing their doubts as to whether they were using the right formula for their prayer or spell. Both were seeing their beliefs ricochet off reality's hardened wall and hit them square between the eyes.

It's a dilemma people have when they only see two explanations for unanswered prayer. They either believe there's something wrong with their faith or there is something wrong with them.

The cutter thought there was something wrong with her, so she kept cutting. But as the Christian woman unfolded her story, I heard her explore a third option.

"Maybe," she said, "there's still a way to accept what's happening to me and to enjoy the life that I have remaining. Maybe that's a better miracle than what my parents are praying for."

Something happened at that point in the conversation. She wondered aloud what it might be like if she lived her faith, not as a vehicle for getting what she wanted, but as a way to unlock the story of who she was. Perhaps it was possible, she thought, that God wouldn't be manipulated through a formula or spell; maybe prayer is a way of healing and expressing our hurts to God.

Sadly, the Wiccan sergeant's path led her to some poor conclusions about her self-image — those that would lead to her transfer to a mental health facility.

The Apostolic woman, however, went home with a much improved spiritual health. She finally saw a God whose love isn't canceled out by our disappointments in Him. She saw a God who promises to remain present in our pain, even when things may seem out of control.

Faith in the Afterlife

The fourth component of faith is a belief in the life that follows, often called the afterlife. However, people of faith often deny just how close they are to that afterlife. Take for example the day I walked though our hospital on my patient rounds when my pager diverted me to the Emergency Department.

Moments later I arrived to watch the doctors compressing the chest of a 60-something-year-old man.

The charge nurse standing in the door redirected my attention toward a family in our consultation area. In a room the size of walk-in closet, I found the patient's wife perched on a chair's edge with a manila folder in her lap.

I introduced myself to the woman and told her the doctors were performing CPR on her husband. I assured her we were doing everything possible to save his life.

"No," she said. "He doesn't want that."

"Pardon me?"

The woman answered by pulling an Advanced Directive (Living Will) from her file. The bilingual paperwork detailed her husband's terminal cancer and specified that he didn't want to be resuscitated or kept alive by artificial means.

I excused myself and darted across the hall and into the hectic trauma room where I delivered the time-sensitive information.

"Doctor!" I said, "Our patient is a 'DNR' (do not resuscitate). The patient's wife brought the paperwork."

After some quick clarification, the doctor halted her resuscitation efforts and pronounced the patient dead.

A few minutes later, I escorted the man's family into the room where he'd died. While his family whispered their goodbyes in Spanish, I couldn't help but respect a man who had pushed his life right up to the last moment and then released it with a final breath.

However, there are those who don't believe it's necessary to push a terminal disease right up to the last possible moment. They are people like 29-year-old Oregonian Brittany Maynard.

Maynard was the newlywed diagnosed with terminal brain cancer. While fate chose the disease, Maynard chose the following Saturday as the day she'd die.

By all accounts, Maynard was not suicidal, or even depressed. She simply hoped to avoid the insufferable days of her disease. She was very clear that she wanted a "good death," pain-free and with some dignity to spare.

As a hospital chaplain, I'm sympathetic with people like Maynard. I've watched scores of people die painful and undignified deaths. I've seen doctors order excruciating and invasive tests on terminal patients for seemingly little purpose than avoiding the obvious. My observations led me to consider three issues about euthanasia.

First, physical pain is often the biggest fear of the terminally ill. Gratefully, medicine continues to improve efforts to help people die pain-free. Still, we need more weapons in the arsenal of pain control — methods that don't put people in a coma or covertly kill them.

Second, unless you're facing a painful demise, I think it's nearly impossible to judge the morality of Maynard's choice. In fact, I'm not sure how any one of us would decide differently. Nevertheless, hopelessness cannot excuse the failure to search for more options.

Finally, I believe that as people of faith, we need to move away from the notion that assisted suicide (or any suicide) is an unforgivable sin. Maynard's choice doesn't send her to hell — far from it. Christian Scripture promises, "Nothing can separate us from the love of God." I suppose that's why, as the family gathered for their bilingual goodbyes in our emergency room, they said, "Vaya con Dios." Go with God.

I watch people die almost every day in my job as a hospital chaplain. Few are as prepared for it as my ER patient with an Advance Directive. Actually, I think you might be shaken if you saw how those deaths are painfully delayed because the family never took the time to have an understanding of the patient's wishes.

For example, an 82-year-old farmer came to our ER with a failing heart. Doctors twice restarted his heart and transferred him to ICU on a ventilator. After a few days, his doctors saw little hope and asked our palliative care team to talk to the family about options.

Palliative care is a philosophy that encourages quality of life over quantity of life. The Mayo Clinic website says the approach "…offers pain and symptom management and emotional and spiritual support [in the] face of a chronic, debilitating or life-threatening illness."

Our team, composed of a chaplain, nurse, social worker and doctor, met with the farmer's three grown children in a conference room. For 20 minutes, the doctor outlined two choices.

First, the family could ask us to do "everything." Meaning, if the farmer's heart stopped, we would do chest compressions and electric shock. If he stopped breathing, we'd put a tube down his throat and help him breath. And if needed, we'd even insert the breathing tube through an incision in the windpipe. Later we might add a feeding tube through the stomach.

"But for what purpose? To make him better?" the doctor said. "He won't get better."

The doctor was voicing what our team was thinking – namely that the patient should meet two requirements for this option. He has to want it and it has to be helpful – neither was true.

The second option presented was for the family to allow the natural process of dying to take place with dignity and without pain.

The family studied their laps as they insisted they couldn't make that decision. "Please," they said, "just keep doing everything. We are leaving this in God's hands."

The doctor turned a glance in my direction, like a soccer player heading the ball to a player who had a clearer shot at the goal.

I cleared my throat as I considered my best approach.

"Leaving it up to God" in this context is often an expression of procrastination rather than faith. The saying conveys a fear that God can't answer the tough questions. It quickly becomes a religious coin toss between denial and faith.

But worst of all, it highlights a contradiction: If we're really "leaving it up to God," why do we need these machines to keep the ball in play? If we truly left it up to God, we wouldn't be playing tug of war with the patient's soul.

It was this second point I stressed the most. "Might God's will also be expressed in your father's dignified death just as it was in his venerable life?"

They looked further under the table as the oldest repeated the request. "Please do everything possible, including CPR."

In an article that went viral in 2011, "How Doctors Die," Dr. Ken Murray says this is no option at all. He says "when a patient suffers from severe illness, old age, or a terminal disease, the odds of a good outcome from CPR are infinitesimal, while the odds of suffering are overwhelming. Poor knowledge and misguided expectations lead to a lot of bad decisions."

Sadly, this case was the family's misguided expectations of God. The farmer endured two more weeks and three chest-pounding episodes of CPR. Finally, on day 15, the family truly turned it over to God, life support was removed and the farmer was welcomed into the green fields of heaven.

As people of faith, we testify that we are prepared and that we know what is after this life. Still we resist. The majority of the patients I meet are in denial much like someone I'll call Mr. Stanley, a 76-year-old Korean veteran I met in the VA hospital three years ago.

Stanley's heart was failing, and he was struggling to find breath as his tearful wife of 50 years kept trading glances between him and his heart monitor. At some point, she asked me to bless him. I thought back to my Baptist upbringing. We usually only prayed for the sick; blessing someone was not a rite we practiced.

However, because I work hard to bring a nonjudgmental presence and deliver what people need in their moment of crisis, I wrote a blessing for him. I began by placing one hand on Stanley's shoulder and holding the other open before me, as if I was expecting something to be placed in it.

"May God place you in his hand and hold you there.

May he pull you close to his heart."

Cupping my outstretched hand over my own heart, I added:

> "May you know the beating of God's heart.
> May your heart match the rhythm of his heart.
> May his spirit fill your lungs with the healing breath of life.
> May you know the calling of his direction.
> May you hear his voice and find a peace that passes all
>   understanding.
> I pronounce this blessing on you in the name of the Father,
>   son and Holy Spirit."

As I looked across at Mrs. Stanley, I saw a certainty forming on her face that wasn't previously there. She and I both knew that God had brought some dignity of purpose to the moment.

My blessing wasn't terribly creative, but it brought power in the lives of Mr. and Mrs. Stanley that really can't be disputed.

Given the opportunity to express their fear of death, most people become rather logical. This is something I saw a few years back when a psychologist, a social worker and a doctor accompanied me into the hospital room of an 84-year-old Korean War Vet who I remember as Ken. The doctor, a consulting physician, introduced us as the palliative care team for the VA Hospital.

Ken's wife of 51 years stood to shake our hands with a self-assured grip. The woman, likely in her seventies, had the well-heeled look of a senior model. Ken, the victim of multiple strokes, did little to greet us, preferring instead the revolving wheel of a TV game show.

With introductions made, we pushed our chairs into a semicircle around Ken's bed. Our psychologist, a ponytailed man pushing 60, spoke first. Had her husband been able to dress, feed and bathe himself? Did she think he had much understanding of what was going on with his body?

"No" to all those questions.

The doctor then assumed control of the meeting by picking up her stethoscope. She was an athletic woman who'd had some luck cheating her 50s with youthful blue eyes and a pixie cut. She bent over Ken, searching his expression for understanding, but she saw little to indicate that he was aware of his surroundings.

"He really needs a feeding tube," the doctor concluded.

"Then let's do that," the wife said.

Actually there were few options left for the old vet. He'd had multiple hospitalizations and suffered several recent bouts of pneumonia. Each illness was followed by weeks in a rehabilitation facility in the San Francisco Bay area.

With great sensitivity, the doctor told the woman that even with the feeding tube, Ken would likely aspirate his saliva. In addition, he'd have to be restrained or heavily sedated because stroke-induced confusion would cause Ken to pull out the tube.

"Is this the way your husband wanted to live his later years?" the psychologist asked.

"No," she said. "I suppose it really isn't."

"Sounds like he values the quality of his life," I reflected.

She nodded. "He knows that heaven awaits."

The hour-long meeting finished when Ken's wife agreed to let us implement "comfort care measures."

Comfort care means that every person taking care of Ken would adopt a new goal — one designed not to make Ken get better, but to make him feel better. Our goal shifted to helping him live as well as possible for as long as possible. With the help of social work, psychology and chaplaincy, we would now care for Ken's whole person.

The real reason behind this difficult meeting was that Ken, like many people, had failed to discuss crucial questions with his loved ones prior to arriving on his deathbed.

Those questions are contained in the advance directive, (sometimes called a living will). An advance directive is the document that directs the doctors to follow the wishes of patients who are unable to speak for themselves.

If you don't have a written directive, or you haven't appointed someone who can confidently speak for you, then doctors will be obligated to do everything possible — even if "everything" means a painful delay of your death.

Ken was well loved by family and fellow vets, but the truth is that a well-written advance directive could have eased the burden on his family and ensured that he'd have spent his final days with the dignity of his choosing.

If you don't have an advance directive, I urge you to get started today. More information on advance directives, and state-specific advance directive documents to download, are available at caringinfo.org.

Sometimes our denial of death can sound downright religious in our resistance to the end. Early in my chaplain work, I got a phone call from Grace, the nurse manager in our intensive care unit. In an impatient tone that fell short of her namesake quality, she tersely asked, "Chaplain, what are you doing at 2 p.m.?"

"Uh . . ." Caught off guard, my afternoon schedule suddenly vanished from my memory. As chaplain for a Houston hospital in the early 1990s, my days stayed pretty full, but at that moment, I couldn't remember what I was doing in the next minute, let alone several hours later.

"We have an end-of-life conference with a family. Can you make it?" Frustrated by the lengthy use of an ICU bed, Grace had called the conference to discuss continuing life support for a seventy-five-year-old male stroke victim who had shown no sign of brain activity for sixty days.

"Life support" is a misnomer. At times like this, it should be called "mechanical maintenance." This man wasn't being *supported*; he was being *preserved*. Yet despite those efforts, his body was literally decaying. Typically, most TV-watching Americans describe the process of discontinuing life support as "pulling the plug." They picture a nurse grimly yanking twenty tubes from every orifice or throwing a big switch somewhere that turns off all the electronic apparatuses, sending the patient's room into a quiet hush except for the flat-line hum of the monitor. Actually, it's far less dramatic, involving the slow turning of a few knobs. Done properly, it's usually a peaceful process.

When this family showed up in the conference room, it was quickly apparent that their hearts weren't anywhere near ready for our discussion. This family was "claiming a miracle." They didn't care what anyone said. They were claiming that their father would rise from his deathbed in three days. That was their definition of a miracle, defined and customized.

Shifting the conversation, I asked them what it might be like if they redefined what a miracle meant in this situation. What would a miracle look like, I asked, if they allowed the frame to be removed from their picture of God—if they accepted that the mysterious and unlimited workings of God might produce a miracle that differed from the one they had in mind?

Consider Jesus' example, and you'll see that even he was sometimes uncomfortable with the use of miracles. He didn't intend them as something that would prove the existence of God. He told one group of scoffers that even if he were to raise someone from the dead, they still wouldn't believe. The fact is, we may learn as much from studying Jesus' *avoidance* of miracles on certain occasions as we do by reading how and when he did perform them. For instance, at Calvary he was taunted by people who demanded that he come down from the cross. "He saved others," they sneered, "but he can't save himself!" (Matthew 27:42). It never occurred to them that a miracle was occurring even his closest followers couldn't see (although Jesus had told them it would happen).

Like those disciples, we, too, often overlook the real miracles. Maybe, while we're waiting and watching for one preconceived miracle to happen, something else happens but we fail to see the miraculous in it.

For instance, maybe the true miracle isn't always going to be that Dad survives cancer but that his prodigal children come back into his life. Perhaps the real miracle will not be a baby's survival after a difficult birth but that somehow she will introduce a presence of God to her family or even to hospital staffers.

Miracles aren't always about getting something back; sometimes they are about finding a fuller appreciation for what you have left when that something is taken away. Maybe the true miracle isn't always going to be about saving the world but about gaining new appreciation for a piece of it.

During the week following the end-of-life conference (in which the family did finally agree to discontinue life support), I saw at least two small miracles. That father didn't walk out of our hospital, no, but three sisters found agreement in prayer as they united at their father's bedside and gave him permission to walk into the arms of a waiting God. That was the first small miracle. And the second and more lasting miracle was that the sisters discovered an infinite God whom they could not control.

And in my experience, knowing a God whom you cannot control is the first step toward knowing that God is in control.

While Heaven my wait, my lunch will not. I was on the hunt for fried chicken during my lunch hour from the hospital where I worked as a pediatric chaplain a few years back when my cell phone rang.

Because my policy was to never, ever, give my cell number to a patient's family, I was totally oblivious to the likelihood of a serious call during lunch.

I cheerfully answered the phone.

"Chaplain, where is he?"

"Sarah?" I asked.

"I mean . . ." Sarah stammered. "Eric's in Heaven, right?"

Sarah was the mother of a little boy who had died in our hospital a few weeks prior. For some reason — I didn't really know why — there was something special about this close-knit family that caused me to make an exception about my cell phone rule.

"Yes, I feel certain that he is in heaven," I declared, shifting gears from fast-food to food for thought.

When I asked her to tell me more about what was going on, she told me she was having nightmares about her son smothering. Her sobs continued and churned an ocean of grief. The swells came through the phone like waves threatening to drown both swimmer and rescuer.

Then she asked something that can't possibly be answered definitively by anyone on this side of the celestial.

"What was it like for him after he died? What's he feeling now?"

The Bible contains many references about heaven, but Sarah was not looking for biblical authority, she was looking to share in another parent's deepest hope. Living inside a pain that was raw and brutal, she was trying to make it through her personal hell on earth, one day at a time, one prayer at a time, one phone call at a time.

I tried my best to answer her question, but given my current whereabouts I opted to add a bit more through a later e-mail.

"I don't know for sure what Heaven's like," I wrote. "The Bible tells me God prepared it as a 'place not made with hands,' so it's probably more than we could ever imagine. And if it's made by God, then Heaven must be made of the best of us, of who we are, of all our hearts can collectively imagine.

"Sarah, you cared for Eric every hour of every day for eight years. Your love formed a cocoon of Heaven for him right here on Earth. God has done no less for Eric by creating an eternal Heaven designed by a mother's love and a father's care.

"When I think of Eric in Heaven, I see him in a place where his lungs are filled with the freshest air from the most pristine mountain peaks. It is a place where he needn't struggle to find his legs. He can walk and run and jump. He can dance with butterflies and sing with angels.

"He can talk and hear and understand. He knows the joy of a million rainbow waterfalls. He knows a father who loves him and is filled with the presence of his mother's lullaby to comfort him."

After sending the e-mail, I resolved to amend my phone policy about not giving my personal number to patients.

God knows who needs to talk and when. I think God knew I needed to talk to Sarah as much as she needed to talk to me.

So, God mysteriously gave her the number — via my big mouth.

Now, I have a new cell number policy: "Never, never, never give a patient your personal phone number, unless of course, it's God's idea."

Denying your need to grieve is just as bad as denying the inevitability of death. As a hospital chaplain, I'm often asked what "normal" grief looks like. For instance, a staff member may notice a wailing hospital visitor and ask, "Is that normal?" or a weeping family member will ask, "Is it normal to be so angry?"

Few people have done a better job identifying the grief process than Elisabeth Kübler-Ross. Her 20th-century research named five grief components: denial, anger, bargaining, depression and acceptance.

Ten years ago, I watched those characteristics unfold in the email of a 28-year-old mother that I'll call Alicia. The email expressed "unanswered questions and concerns" after her baby daughter, Sarah, died in our hospital. While I can't print the entire email, I want you to notice the normal grief stages in the excerpts below.

She begins her email in denial. "I am second guessing what more could have been done. I am still not 100% clear what exactly happened. ... Even though I saw Sarah and held her as she died ... it just still has not sunk in."

The letter also expressed anger at the staff for not calling the grieving family in the days after the funeral. Alicia remembers, "We had everyone's support, and then my daughter died and all the support ended."

The letter's bargaining paragraphs teeter between belief and doubt. First she says, "It provides me comfort in believing Sarah's in heaven and with God." But then she challenges her own faith by suggesting that heaven could have been "started by grievers who needed some solace in believing that there is more after death, that believing that it exists just helps people cope."

Then, she stumbles back into believing: "Because to think that heaven doesn't exist and that Sarah doesn't live on ... is more than I can handle, more than I can truly bear."

Her depression stains the email with tears, crying: "Being in constant sadness and turmoil is such a difficult place to be. Sometimes, I am just not sure what to do to get through this; it is so painful. Sometimes I just want to hide from the pain, because it is more ... than I have the strength to take on."

She closes her email introducing the notion of acceptance. "But yet here I am, still moving forward ... a day further than yesterday, so I must have the strength to do it. ... I will get past this time and I will see better times, but of course I will never be the same. I will never forget her, and she will always be a part of me and there will always be a part of me that died along with her.

Alicia ends her letter by saying: "I have been lucky enough to dream about my daughter. ... One in particular, my daughter was about the size and age when she died, she was sitting in my lap and just as happy as can be, smiling at me with this big opened-mouth grin."

Alicia began her letter with "unanswered questions and concerns." While I don't remember my exact reply, I avoid the questionable answers that are often given in the name of religion. Answers like, "God needed your child more than you," or "God won't give you more than you can handle."

If there's anything I know from being a hospital chaplain, it's that I have few answers. Instead, I find that when I invite people to speak the unspeakable and ask the unanswerable questions, they begin to discover the answers that fit their needs – not mine. And at the end of the day, their answers are likely to be the most normal ones to be found.

Hell if I know much about hell. However, I was raised by a Southern Baptist pastor who spun some dramatic sermons about hell. He often used il-lustrations from people he was trying to detour from their road to perdition.

I remember how he'd lean his 6-foot frame over the pulpit and smooth the air with the dismissive gesture of downturned palms. "People often tell me, 'Preacher, I want to go to hell, because that's where my beer-drinking friends will be.'"

Then my father cued his congregation with a headshake until rippling chuckles announced that parishioners were ready to hear how he'd out-smarted his skeptics.

"I tell them, 'When you get to hell, your friends will desert you.'" Then, mixing bass into his punch-line logic, he said "And that'll be your hell."

During my 30 years of ministry, I've encountered similar logic, but I believe my father's stories illustrated people's misunderstanding of heaven more than they did their understanding of hell.

They saw heaven as a place where they'd be forced to behave. It then became a simple choice. They'd rather ditch the saints in heaven and go to hell with "a better class of losers" – as Randy Travis says.

That kind of thinking reminds me of a disheveled man who recently came into my office.

"I'm dying," he told me. "I have cancer throughout my body."

"I'm sorry," I managed to say.

"Don't be," he said. "Just pray that I'll make better choices during my last months."

"OK," I said, accepting the hand he offered. "I'll pray."

I prayed for everything he'd requested: forgiveness for his rough life and a chance to reconcile with his family.

When I finished, I heard him clear his throat. "Lord! You know me." I wasn't expecting the addendum, but I bowed my head again.

"I know that I can't have sex or alcohol in heaven," he said. I opened one eye to see if this man was just having fun with his chaplain, but I knew he was serious. "And Lord, that's going to suck big time! But I still want to go."

I was impressed. I wasn't sure I'd ever met a man who was willing to give up so much to see God.

Now I'm not a theologian. I'm not even on the Celestial Entertainment Committee, but whoever taught this man that following God is about giving up his joy was dead wrong.

The good news is that God created all of us, and we will return to him one day. Heaven will become this man's repatriation where he will be restored to his country of origin. He will shed his notions of what he has to give up and will encounter a being much more loving and accepting than anyone had ever dared to tell him about.

My father always preached that most eternal questions would have to be answered in the "sweet by-and-by" – which I know is a major disappointment to those of you who are still wondering whether there'll be sex in heaven or beer in hell.

Grieving is normal, but the Bible does urge us not to grieve as those who have no hope. Such was the example of a man dying in one of our hospital beds last year. He was nearly 90, so he was definitely old enough to die. However, the question his family was asking when I walked into his room was whether he was ready to die.

"Hi, I'm Chaplain Norris," I said to the octogenarian.

"A chaplain?" he asked with the lilt of delighted surprise. Then with a toothless smile he added, "Hi, Norris."

"Hello, Sir," I said, hinting at his naval years in the Greatest Generation.

It was the type of conversation I don't have too often in my role as a hospital chaplain or even as a military chaplain. It was different because our patient was lucid enough to see what lay ahead while still able to acknowledge where he was now. In hospital language, he was "oriented to time and place."

His children and friends surrounded his bed as one of them began humming a favored family hymn. Soon, the rest of his visitors took their cue and music filled the sacred space. As their lyrics spilled into the open hallway, our staff gathered for the moment we knew was coming.

Some glad morning when this life is o'er,
I'll fly away;
To a home on God's celestial shore,
I'll fly away

A slanted smile found its way through the man's pained expressions as he made an attempt to join the chorus.

I'll fly away, Oh Glory
I'll fly away;
When I die, Hallelujah, by and by,
I'll fly away.

More humming. More quiet and then a request.

"Will you say a prayer, Chaplain?" asked his daughter.

The invitation to pray for a dying patient brings unspoken questions: What shall I pray? Do I pray that the patient will live a few more years? Or do I pray that his dying comes without pain?

In a clinical setting these prayerful questions are often rendered: What would the patient want? Aggressive care? Or a painless passing? His family reluctantly decided to pray for the latter.

In my prayer, I brought the words of the psalmist to reassure his family that there was no place that their dad could go without the comforting presence of God:

> "Where can I go from your Spirit?
> Where can I flee from your presence?
> If I go up to the heavens, you are there;"

My prayer prompted a question from a family member that I hear almost weekly in the hospital — not a question really, more a confession looking for absolution.

"I feel so selfish," they often say. "I don't want him to die, but I know he hurts too much to stay here."

It's a plea I frequently answer with some reassurance. "No, that's not selfish at all. That's just a good indication of how much you loved him and how much he loved you."

The real truth in the moment was that their dad had earned the privilege to die in these supportive surroundings. Committed to the woman he'd married, he'd raised his children and loved them with his last breath. He'd watched his wife die the previous year and now he was the last to go through death's portal. He was ready to die and he expressed no regrets.

I hope I can face death with the kind of resilience I saw in this dying vet. It was the same resilience I saw in a particular patient I met on another day in the VA hospital where I served as a per diem chaplain.

The old vet was sitting on the edge of his bed, hunched over his considerable stomach, studying the floor tiles when I walked in.

"Hello," I called as I walked into his darkened room. "I'm Norris, the hospital chaplain." He dialed a smile onto his liver-spotted face and replied with an upturned tone of recognition.

"Hello, Norris!" I took study of his expressive blue eyes and the swirling tumbleweed of hair atop a balding head, but felt no flash of recognition. Still, with a lingering air of familiarity, he invited me onto the bedside chair like an old friend who'd come to visit. "I'm so glad you came, Chaplain," he said. "I'm a pastor, too."

It turned out I didn't know him, but I knew the pastoral pitch and ministerial mannerisms. I knew him. I was looking at myself 25 years from now. "Are you retired now?" I asked, an unintentional reference to his weighty encumbrance.

"Are we ever really retired?" His mention of "we" felt like a club handshake. "I guess not," I said. "We definitely signed up for the duration." "That's right. Ours is a lifelong service."

During the next half hour, he unfolded 50 years, beginning with his marriage to his college sweetheart. Together, they started a church as well as a family. She birthed a baby girl one year and a son the next. However, not long after birth, their son started turning blue. They called for an ambulance, but it came too late.

"It was congenital," he told me. The tears were now leaking from his reddened eyes, taking their evacuation route over bulging cheeks. A problem in the baby's heart shattered the heart of his parents. "It was all so long ago," he said.

His tone became apologetic, as if mystified by the source of his tears. "You cry because it happened out of order. You're grieving the loss of potential, for what could have been." He nodded.

"There's an old Chinese proverb," I said. "True Happiness is: Grandfather dies. Father dies. Son dies. Grandson dies."

Yet, even as I spoke, he was waving a dismissive hand. It seemed likely he'd heard this before and even more likely he'd said it to himself. Then, as if announcing another chapter of his autobiography, he said, "There's more. "The cancer.

"My firstborn," he stuttered. "She died when she was just 39."

"You lost two children?" Mine was half question and half-hearted indictment toward our celestial employer for expecting a man to remain in ministry after such tragedy.

I guess he caught my meaning because he said, "I'll be in heaven ten thousand years before I'll ever understand why."

I sat in silence with that observation. The old preacher knew the answers were so complex that ten thousand years of deliberation couldn't bring any real understanding.

I suppose I could have reminded him that God "… causes his sun to rise on the evil and the good, and sends rain on the righteous and the unrighteous" (Matthew 5:45), but he likely knew that. He didn't need more verses; he needed to know that God still heard his pain.

I reached for his hand, asked if we could tell this to God. He nodded. We prayed. We cried. Just as he was wiping his last tear, his wife came into the room.

He concluded his story by adding that he was now serving as Pastor Emeritus and advising the younger pastors. I guess he was right. Serving God is an endless calling, but doing so with such a gaping wound to the soul brings to mind nothing short of the divine.

7

BUILDING LASTING RESILIENCE
WITH FORGIVENESS

There is no way to remain resilient in this life without being on both the giving and receiving end of forgiveness. However, I don't know about you, but I occasionally get hung up on that part of the Lord's Prayer that encourages us to pray, "Forgive us our trespasses as we forgive those who trespass against us."

Forgiveness is hard even for a chaplain, but I can't possibly conceive what it was like for Amon Goeth depicted in Steven Spielberg's 1993 movie "Schindler's List."

The movie is the true story of the sadistically cruel, Auschwitz camp commandant, Amon Goeth. In a poignant scene, Commandant Goeth randomly sights Jewish prisoners through his riflescope and kills them for the tiniest infraction in their daily chores.

Schindler saw this sadistic practice as Goeth's quest for power. To slow the killing, Schindler conned Goeth into trying a different path to power.

"You can be such a big man," he coaxed, "by forgiving these foolish Jews for their mistakes. Instead of shooting them, say 'I forgive you.' You are the great Amon Goeth! What Aryan nobility you could show!"

Goeth thinks about it for a few days. Then, he suddenly appears amidst his terrified captives offering this haphazardly pronouncement: "I forgive you. Ah, yes, I forgive you."

Of course, the absurdity of the scene is that Goeth lacks the spiritual power to either condemn or forgive. Nevertheless, Schindler's point is profound — the power to forgive is ultimate power. Schindler knew that "I forgive you" is easily the most powerful pronouncement on the planet.

If you don't believe me, check out the biblical story in Mark 2 where some friends of a paralyzed man bring him to a home where Jesus is speaking.

At first, the crowds prove impenetrable. But his determined friends raise the paralytic onto the roof of the home, punch a hole, and then lower the suffering soul into the middle of the crowd surrounding Jesus.

Impressed by the bold belief of the friends, Jesus gives a startling response to the paralytic. "Friend, I forgive your sins."

The religious leaders found Jesus' proclamation as preposterous as the Jews probably found Goeth's statement. They ask the crowd, "Who does he (Jesus) think he is? That's blasphemous talk! God, and only God, can forgive sins."

Jesus challenges his detractors by posing a comparison.

"Which is simpler: to say 'I forgive your sins,' or to say 'Get up and start walking'?" The syntax of his question implies the answer he expected — forgiveness is much harder.

For a time, pseudo-forgiveness came easy to the Nazi commandant. He delighted himself in his new power to forgive. However, his satisfaction was short-lived because he was only using forgiveness to manipulate people for his amusement.

We've all met this type of person. They don't use a gun like Goeth did, but they manipulate us by creating a sense of indebtedness to them. They forgive us only so they can get what they need.

The forgiveness offered by Jesus bestowed the power to heal and to restore all who were involved, not just the forgiver.

How did the story end? I like the way The Message puts it — "Just so it's clear that I'm . . . authorized to do either . . ." He spoke directly to the paraplegic: "Get up. Take your bedroll and go home." Without a moment's hesitation, he did it.

Then the passage says: "They rubbed their eyes, incredulous—and then praised God, saying, "We've never seen anything like this!""

Such is the power of genuine forgiveness. Try it.

An unforgiving spirit can be haunting. I know. For a long time I was haunted by some very dead issues. I found myself so troubled, that I started talking to the dead.

"Wait a minute!" you say? "I knew this was a spiritual book, but I didn't think it was THAT kind of spirit."

No worries. I'm not talking about séances; I'm talking about the way we tend to resurrect issues and hurts that are dead and gone.

In this area, I have occasionally played the medium.

One afternoon, four years ago, I had been flirting with some of these dead issues – hurts that I couldn't seem to release.

These hurts came nearly as audible voices, and when my wife overheard me conversing with them, she challenged me to call my pastor.

But wait. I was a pastor, so whom should a pastor call? I called my life pastor, my father-in-law, Wil. Over the next few days, he challenged me to make some time in which I could work on releasing these hurts.

"How?" I asked.

Wil answered that question a week later when he showed up at our home with my mother-in-law. He brought my wife and I into our living room and we formed a circle. From that circle, he read something that changed my life. It was called, "**A Litany for Our Deepest Hurts**."

Here's how it reads:

Leader: Because there are pains that do not heal as physical pain does with time, surgery, or medication, we are engaged in this spiritual covenant in anticipation – now or soon – of eventual healing of our spirits.

Response: I accept and enter this covenant as if I were beginning a brand new journey in life.

Leader: The deeper the hurt, the longer the journey, whether in minutes, hours or days, to that healing destination brought about by forgiveness and release.

Response: I promise to move in that direction. I may not move as fast as you think I should, but today or daily I will release and surrender either all or some part of this cumbersome weight.

Leader: These hurts have many names such as bushwhacked, waylaid, back-stabbed, slandered, deceived, etc., and none hurt like that received from a perceived friend.

Response: I will cease giving it a name and simply reject anything in my mind and spirit that is counterproductive to what God has planned for me.

Leader: Ceasing to dwell on this matter is not a matter of weakness, for it will free your time and mind. Therefore, if you are willing to stop looking back and instead face a forward direction, then our mighty God will be better able to bless and direct a forward-moving life.

Response: Because I know you are right, I hereby give up to God my so-called "rights" I have attached to my hurts, knowing He will deal with those involved while also leading me "in the paths of righteousness for His name's sake."

Since then, I've shared this litany in dozens of churches in my talks across the US. It's also become my most requested reprint with many fellow strugglers. While no one has found it to be a magic pill, most have found it useful as a strong first step toward deliberately ceasing to call on these dead issues.

As for myself, I continue to remember the litany as a daily touchstone, reminding me as does my Al-Anon friend, "Do you want to be right, or righteous?"."

In recent years, we've seen a lot of horrific things on the news in terms of mass shootings. We watch people bring their revenge on police officers and we watch meaningless shootings under the color of authority. Where does it all end? It can only end with forgiveness and grace.

Both are tall orders. But God calls us to walk that path as I discovered years ago when a father brought his 3-year-old, blond-haired boy to our Houston hospital. The dad told us that he had been "horsing around" with his son when the boy suddenly began vomiting. A few minutes after their arrival, doctors pronounced the boy dead.

The police came and the questions followed. Dad and mom were in the same profession — stripping. While she'd been dancing at the club, dad says he gave his son a playful stomach punch.

In the midst of that, I was his chaplain; the guy who sat with a tearful dad when mom bolted through our automatic door, echoing my thoughts with her words: "You son of a b—-! What have you done?"

Over the next few hours, I escorted each of the family members into the room where the little boy lay. They don't get much cuter than this kid, and I supported the grandparents as they grieved over the loss of a grandson and the mom over the loss of her child.

But when the dad straightened his grief-bent frame and asked me to take him to his son, I had to ask myself how in God's name could I support an animal that did this to his own son? What was he grieving?

I took him anyway. As he stood at the gurney, confronted with the results of his "play," he wept. He was sorry in his own depraved way — sorry he didn't have a son anymore, sorry he ruined so many lives, and no doubt, sorry he was going to prison.

He needed a chaplain at that moment. And while I definitely did not feel like being that chaplain, God didn't ask me how I felt about it.

Neither did God ask Edwin Zeiders, pastor of St. Paul's Methodist Church at State College, Pa. In 2008, Zeiders sat in court with his parishioner of 30 years, former Penn State assistant football coach and accused child molester, Jerry Sandusky.

Zeiders put words to his role when he appeared before reporters to say, "We continue to define the local congregation as a people of love and restoration, while giving witness and an endless stream of mercy from our Lord and the forgiveness that opens the doorway to new life."

There's a time to rage against injustice, but there's also a moment when God calls us to see all the victims. Both the father I met in the hospital and Sandusky blame their predicament on harmless horseplay, which tells me that they are victims of their own self-deception. These men need a pastor, and their victims need our prayers.

Zeiders set the bar high in his statement, but I would soon see the bar raised even higher.

The loud weeping penetrated the walls of our hospital chapel so much so that I could hear them in my office next door. At first, it didn't seem that unusual. I often heard pulsing sobs that were uncontainable by the chapel wall.

I stood, pushing my chair away from my desk. I wondered what I would find this time. Would it be a mother crying for her child in surgery?

Would it be someone bargaining with God to save an alcoholic partner? Or would it be a community member praying for an errant child?

I'd seen all of these.

I opened the chapel door to see a petite woman nearly drowning in her tears. I couldn't make out all of her words, but it was clear she was sorry about something.

What was she sorry for? Something about her daughter. Was she sick? In an accident? Newly diagnosed with a terminal disease?

Wait. Was this the woman a nurse had earlier described in whispered tones? Was this the woman who brought her 6-year-old daughter to the hospital after beating her into a coma?

It was, and she was crying, begging God for forgiveness.

So, in the midst of her tears, I delivered the hospital chaplain's version of the Miranda rights. "I'm a hospital employee," I said, "I can be subpoenaed to testify about whatever is said here — even in the chapel."

A few minutes later, I wasn't surprised when the chapel door opened revealing two detectives anxious to talk to her.

What did surprise me over the next few hours and days, however, was the presence of people from her church Bible study group.

It seemed to me that this woman likely had committed an unpardonable sin. Even Jesus condemned anyone who would harm a child saying that "would be better for him to have a large millstone hung around his neck and be drowned in the depths of the sea."

I was ready to drown this woman myself.

So how was it that this church could provide such a caring presence, let alone promise the presence of unconditional love voiced by a perfect God?

Yet there they stood. Quiet. Admittedly shocked, but nevertheless, they formed a presence without a voiced judgment.

I couldn't help but wonder: Did their presence bring love? Or were they over-the-line dysfunctional?

People are so imperfect in their love. They're capable of loving an errant spouse, yet sometimes incapable of loving their children. They love one parent, but not the other. They love animals, but not the homeless.

We possess an incredible ability to compartmentalize our love and then deliver it in the most inhospitable environments. We can love the most unlovable things.

I spent several weeks at the girl's bedside, watching her father wipe her drool and search her vacant eyes for the girl he once knew. And I have to tell you, I'll never find much love for this woman; I don't expect that you would either.

If this church could still show a loving and caring presence toward that woman, they must have seen something worth saving that only God could have shown them. The whole thing begged the question: How much more capable is God at loving us? If they could struggle through forgiveness and restoration, how much more can God do?

It's been about four years since I met the woman in the chapel. Since then, the child has died and the woman resides in prison. My hope is that the woman will live with two memories: one of her child and one of God's restorative forgiveness.

Forgiveness can empower your resilience, but I find that even more true in the combat environment.

During my 2009 service as an Air Force chaplain in Iraq, I saw countless examples of heroism. However, the most spiritually heroic act I witnessed was the prayer of a soldier who asked God to forgive the insurgents who had killed his battle buddy.

On Easter morning, 2009, I was the chaplain in the Air Force Field Hospital in Balad, Iraq when three patients were wheeled into our emergency room from a Black Hawk UH-60L helicopter.

The first patient had shrapnel in her right eye and a broken left hand, but seemed OK.

Suddenly she blurts, "I couldn't save him! He's dead, isn't he?"

"Who?" someone asked.

"Our team leader," she said.

In the next few moments, the 98-pound-soldier recalled riding as a medic in a vehicle hit by an EFP (Explosively Formed Projectile) designed to penetrate an armored vehicle. When the half-blinded medic found that her team leader lost a leg, she reached into his hip cavity to pinch the femoral artery closed.

"You did the right thing," our trauma czar told her. "That's what we would have done."

"He kept talking about his wife and unborn child," she added, "But I couldn't maintain my hold."

"Just relax, now. You're safe," said the anesthetist prepping her for surgery. "There's no way to close a hemorrhage that close to the groin."

Soon, after she'd been sedated, I made my way to another soldier with shrapnel injuries to his left leg. As quickly as I offered my help, he voiced a request.

"I want you to pray, chaplain." But there was something in his voice that implied an incomplete sentence. It was as if he was saying, "It's your turn to pray now."

He'd been praying ever since the explosion and, now, with the spent fury of a relay runner he was stretching his prayer baton to me. "I want you to pray that the insurgents will understand that we are trying to make their country better."

"I can do that," I said, giving the naiveté of his battlefield spirituality an assenting nod. "The Bible does say pray for your enemies."

"Yes," he said, "but it says more."

With that cryptic remark, I felt my eyebrows furrow and my neck stiffen as he offered further guidance. "I want you to pray that God will forgive the insurgents that killed my friend."

"What would that kind of prayer sound like?" I asked, reversing our naive roles.

"You know the prayer Jesus said on the cross?" he coaxed as if trying to remind me of a forgotten password, "Father, forgive them, for they know not what they do."

Of course I knew it. It was the prayer Jesus prayed as he, too, bled to death.

The prayer wasn't for himself; it was for the mob who unjustly crucified him.

Jesus had seen his killers not as evil people, but as ignorant ones - ignorant of their complicity in their own downfall. In fact, his prayer echoes through the eons, for me, for the wounded squad, and for the insurgents and for you.

"I think that's a great prayer, Private." I said, still a little unsure of whether I was placating his battlefield shock or mine.

Then, after I said the prayer, but before I allowed my eyes to open, I saw something in the flash of a bloodied collage. I saw the insurgents planting the bomb, the explosion, the medic struggling to treat her squad, the team leader bleeding out, and the private praying for them all.

At that moment, I understood. Our world will remain an unending circle of revenge until we learn, as did this simple and wise soldier, to continually repeat Jesus' prayer. And, as we pray it with all our hearts and souls, it will be answered. If not in this world, then in the next when we hear the promised words of Jesus, "Well done, good and faithful servant."

This soldier's prayer emboldened me to face the resentment I'd harbored for 10 years toward a chaplain colleague. My stubbornness was my real-life enactment of Dr. Seuss' "The Zax."

The Seuss story involves a North-going Zax and a South-going Zax who meet on a narrow trail through the Prairie of Prax. Both refuse to step aside to allow the other to pass. The Zaxes maintain their stubborn standoff until eventually a highway overpass is built around them. The story ends with the Zaxes standing "unbudged in their tracks."

I was the Southern Zax who was "unbudged" in my spiritual tracks. In my revised version, the other guy was the Northern Zax who was not only a stubborn fool, but also a big liar who was out to get me. He was paranoid. He was … blah, blah, blah – so went my amended view of history.

For years, I made showy attempts to deal with my resentment by talking to counselors and praying with pastors. But I always made excuses for not doing what I knew I must do: find my former colleague and confess my part of what now seemed a sum total of banal trivialities.

Five years ago my excuses faded when I accepted a speaking invitation in a city near to my old nemesis. I mustered a small measure of the heroics I'd heard in the soldier's forgiveness prayer and broke my indignant silence. I emailed the chaplain with a meeting request.

Two weeks later, he graciously welcomed me into the church where he served as pastor. Inside his office, we shook hands and sat talking about the things important to everyone: faith, family and purpose. Gradually, the image I had created of him shrunk — but in a good way. It shrunk to the size God made us all.

He told me that he had no memory of the details of those years past. Then he said what I needed to hear: "Whatever I did, I hope you will forgive me."

Then I heard myself saying the words I never thought I'd say: "I hope you will forgive me, too." And just like that, the resentment disintegrated, annihilated by grace, never to return.

There was no idealistic or dramatic ending; we simply shook hands and said our goodbyes. Yet we both found and bestowed the grace we needed. We were no longer Zaxes; we were fellow sojourners working out our salvation in this life.

That young soldier's prayer for forgiveness for his enemies, more than anything else, has taught me that if you want to avoid the path of a Zax, you might want to consider Jesus' advice when he said: "If a fellow believer hurts you, go and tell him — work it out between the two of you. If he listens, you've made a friend." While time may heal all things, I think the tone of Jesus' words favors sooner more than later, and He definitely would not approve of waiting 13 years.

I'm thinking that forgiveness is the heroic choice.

Finally, forgiveness walk hand-in-hand with Christian love. That's something I see everyday as I introduce myself to nearly two dozen patients. Most of them greet me with the friendly respect they normally afford their own pastor or faith leader.

However, there are always a few who meet me with suspicion; they think I've come to convert them, or worse yet, bring bad news.

I try to counter their misguided impressions with a one-two punch. First, I explain that my visit is routine and I'm not carrying any bad news. Then with a reassuring smile I add: "No worries. I'm not here to convert you, baptize you or change your mind about religion."

However, while I'm not the one who delivers bad news, I am the one who sits with the patients as they process it. I'll pull up a chair and help sort out the things that suddenly have become important.

This is often when I hear people recite through what I call their "woulda-coulda-shoulda" list. They say they woulda taken better care of their health; they coulda taken more vacations; they shoulda been a better parent or spouse.

But the biggest "should" that dying patients impose upon their story is that they should have shown more love for people – and in turn received more love.

I believe the kind of love they miss can be found in the famous love chapter from 1 Corinthians 13. Even if you don't read the Bible, you'll recognize the popular chapter from the wedding ceremony.

This past week, as I contemplated the terminal prognosis of a chaplain friend with brain cancer, I sat down and paraphrased the chapter for myself. I'm not nearly as poetic as the Apostle Paul, but I trust you'll find my version meaningful.

Even if I become as persuasive as Martin Luther King,

If I'm as eloquent as John Fitzgerald Kennedy,

Even if I sing opera like Charlotte Church,

If I give the riches of Bill Gates to cure the diseases of the world,

Even if I use the brilliance of Steven Hawking to fathom the secrets of the universe,

Nothing much matters if I don't have love.

I can almost hear a chorus of the dying people I've met. I can feel them grab my collar and pull me close. "Listen," they say in a gravelly, whispering voice. "I'm telling you, if you don't have love, none of it matters. It's all trash."

Do you hear me? If you don't have love, all your efforts to be your best, gain the most, and own it all are garbage. Your arguments are futile. Your life counts for rubbish. Your wisdom is nonsense. Your words are just a pile of stinking manure if you don't have love.

Love is persistent and persevering. It doesn't advertise itself or race to be first in line. It takes no pleasure in the misfortune of others, but sees the real fortune in honest truths.

In the end, the building I occupy will crumble into dust and ashes. But for now, I must focus on these three things in Paul's last verse – "Trust steadily in God, hope unswervingly, love extravagantly. And the best of the three is love." (Message Translation)

Conclusion Thriving in the world since 9/11 has become increasingly difficult. Just surviving seems to be an everyday effort in the wake of mass shootings in America and terrorist actions in Europe. It seems like instead of thriving, we turn all our struggles toward improving the safety of public events.

As a parent and grandparent, I applaud these efforts — to a point.

I have always been a safety advocate. I raised my children with such an awareness of safety that they called me the "safety officer."

As adults, we hear our employers advocate safety. They make us wear hats, helmets and seatbelts.

But no matter what we do, most of us know death can come in the most unexpected ways at unimaginable speed. I learned that lesson in a profound way one afternoon in 1995 when I watched a mother follow her 3-year-old son into our Houston emergency room.

The two of them came by ambulance from a metropolitan subdivision. Their afternoon was spent at the community's beautifully swept tennis court. The gated court was staffed by background-checked employees.

"Can I take off my shoes, Mommy?" the little boy asked.

"Sure," she replied. She wanted him safe, but not overly restricted.

The boy explored his environment as little boys can by kicking at the tennis fence.

This is fun, he must have thought. I'm in a giant playpen with Mommy. I feel safe.

There's no way out and no way for the bad guys to come in. If any trouble came, Mommy was close enough.

Close enough was not fast enough. Her son was standing barefoot on a court dampened by morning rain when he kicked the fence near an improperly grounded outlet.

Some might cynically quote the Christian scripture, "It is appointed unto a man once to die," but the truth is that no one enters a tennis court in expectation of seeing his or her son electrocuted. No one crosses the start line of a race expecting to be legless at the finish.

The good news is that the text admonishes us to live our lives as if we knew death was coming tomorrow. The verse is an encouragement for us to love each person in our lives with the fullness as if we knew it was our last day. It is a verse that helps me, not just survive, but thrive with resilience.

So, I will register for more public events, speak in more community venues, and find communal recreation. With all that has been going on, I will no doubt carry some trepidation to these events. But at the end of day, I know that as close as death can come, I must hold life even closer.

EPILOGUE
STRIVING TOWARD A THRIVING FUTURE

This last word is a personal note to the readers who have been reading my column for several years. Many of your emails are asking how Becky and I will continue to thrive in the future. OK, maybe it's just been my mom asking, but nevertheless I'll tell you too.

First, if there's anything I've learned as a chaplain, it's to never count on the future. I don't want to be like the greedy farmer Jesus described in a parable. This man told himself, "Self, you've done well! You've got it made and can now retire. Take it easy, and have the time of your life!'"

If you know that story, you'll know that God took the old fool's soul on the following morning. With all hopes that I won't become that man, let me share our tentative plans.

Currently, Becky and I are working part time. I visit patients 15 hours a week as a hospice chaplain while she teaches in a job-sharing position three days a week in a year-round public school. That means, when I'm not writing or speaking, we enjoy four-day weekends in the 2013 24' Winnebago View motorhome we purchased in Nov 2015. We are blessed to spend nearly every other weekend exploring our home state of California. Becky also has every fourth month off, so we push our trips into bordering states. We shopped a bargain price four our RV because we plan to resell it in the summer of 2017.

Hopefully, that's when Becky and I will fully retire with pensions from her school and mine from the National Guard. With that, we will shed the old rented mobile home and put our household goods in storage. Then, we will travel far and wide for a few years. Our first stop will be Belgium about four months – then we move to Ecuador.

Ecuador? Are we crazy or what? No, retirement overseas is quite popular. Just Google the subject "overseas retirement" and you'll find Ecuador tops the list of popular places. In fact, you'd be surprised to learn that overseas retirement has become so popular that there are more "undocumented Americans" living in Mexico than we have undocumented Mexicans in the US.

To that end, we went to Ecuador in May 2015 to explore the idea of overseas retirement living. We went 8,000 feet into the cool Andes to find Cuenca Ecuador and meet scores of expats who'd shed the consumerism that dominates American life. We found the cost of living so cheap that most expats were living on less than $2000 a month, putting some of their pensions back into savings.

Many of them sold their belongings and flew to Ecuador with their life essentials in just three suitcases apiece. Then, they rented a home at a fraction of an American home and furnished it with utilitarian essentials from local sources. They are no longer stuck in the revolving door of StuffMart or CostlyCo, so some even build their own furniture or make their own clothing.

No, we haven't completely lost our mind. Remember, we are a military family and we consider ourselves to be immensely resilient. Therefore, we hope to enjoy our military retirement benefit of flying on space-available military aircraft. Eventually, by the end of this decade, we will find our way back home. I'll pull the money from our home sale and hopefully buy a small house with a picket fence in a town that may have a little snow, but rarely a scorching day.

And YES, to answer your last question; I will keep writing my newspaper column as long as my editors keep taking my copy. For, as I've already said, I'm a lot like Dr. Seuss's Sam-I-Am who conquered his aversion to green eggs and ham. That means I will write in a box, with a fox, in a house, with a mouse. I will write here and there ... I will write anywhere.

PS: Contact me in the Spring of 2017 if you want to buy a slightly used motorhome, only driven to church on Sundays by a retired minister and his school teacher wife.

Made in the USA
Columbia, SC
08 October 2018